U0396182

国家中医药管理局中医药国际合作专项（文化类项目）

项目编号：0730–236132ZC0053/02—3

Herbal Tales from the Plant Kingdom

植物王国里的
本草故事

广西壮族自治区药用植物园　编著

Edited by Guangxi Botanical Garden of Medicinal Plants

乐　静　绘

Illustrated by Jing Le

张笑梅　译

Translated by Zhang Xiaomei

广西科学技术出版社

Guangxi Science & Technology Publishing House

·南宁·

Nanning

图书在版编目（CIP）数据

植物王国里的本草故事 / 广西壮族自治区药用植物
园编著；乐静绘；张笑梅译. -- 南宁：广西科学技术
出版社，2024. 6. -- ISBN 978-7-5551-2209-8

Ⅰ. R281.3-49

中国国家版本馆CIP数据核字第2024Y9A546号

ZHIWU WANGGUO LI DE BENCAO GUSHI

植物王国里的本草故事

广西壮族自治区药用植物园　编著　乐静　绘

张笑梅　译

策　　划：赖铭洪	责任编辑：邓　霞　刘晓丽　谢艺文
特邀编辑：李科全	装帧设计：苏　畅　梁　良
责任印制：陆　弟	责任校对：吴书丽

出版人：梁　志　　　　　　　　　　出版发行：广西科学技术出版社

社　　址：广西南宁市东葛路66号　　邮政编码：530022

网　　址：http://www.gxkjs.com　　编辑部：0771-5871673

印　　刷：广西民族印刷包装集团有限公司

开　　本：889 mm × 1240 mm　　1/32

印　　张：7

字　　数：268千字

版　　次：2024年6月第1版

印　　次：2024年6月第1次印刷

书　　号：ISBN 978-7-5551-2209-8

定　　价：68.80元

编委会

Members of the Editorial Board

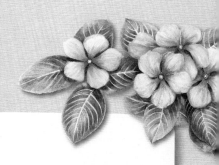

前言

　　中医药是我国优秀传统文化的瑰宝。中草药在为人类防治疾病的同时，还留下了许多具有传奇色彩的有趣故事。编撰本书的目的是普及中草药知识，让小读者们在轻松愉快的故事氛围中学习中医药、了解中医药、接近中医药。

　　本书收载的植物是常见药用植物，编者在编写时，通过生动的植物手绘图，配以植物种名、拉丁学名、趣味小知识或小实验、草药故事等文字，向读者展现了一个缤纷多彩、趣味无穷的中草药世界，还教给读者一些观察和探索中医药知识的方法……这些都有利于培养孩子对中草药的热爱和亲近之情。

　　本书对药用植物的植物种名、药材来源、拉丁学名、性味功效的文字表述，参考了《中国植物志》《中国药典》《中药大辞典》《中草药的故事》等书籍。

　　本书涉及的部分药方的疗效和安全性未经循证医学验证。部分中草药中的有害成分可对人体肾脏、肝脏等造成不可逆损伤。就像神农尝百草、道人仙方疗骨伤等传说故事一样，本书关于中草药的故事亦不可考。因此，本书的内容不作为疾病防治指南，在具体疾病防治过程中，读者务必咨询专业医生。

　　由于编者知识有限，书中难免有错漏之处，欢迎广大读者给予批评指正。

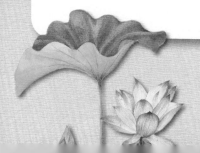

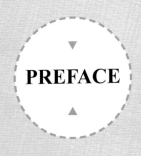

PREFACE

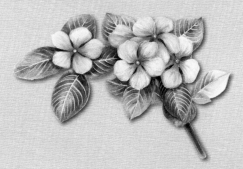

Traditional Chinese medicine (TCM) is the treasure of our excellent traditional culture. Besides preventing and treating diseases, Chinese herbal medicine has been involved in countless captivating stories. This book aims to introduce Chinese herbal medicine through fascinating stories, so that young readers can get to know more about TCM in a joyful way.

Common medicinal plants are listed in this book. It presents readers with a wonderful world about Chinese herbal medicine, featuring vivid hand-drawn plant pictures with their Latin names, fun facts or experiments, and tales. Moreover, readers can learn how to observe and explore those herbs. Therefore, this book is conducive to helping children establish deep relationships with Chinese herbal medicine.

The species name, origins, Latin names, and efficacy of those herbs in this book are partly guided and inspired by the following books: *Flora of China*, *Chinese Pharmacopoeia*, *The Dictionary of Traditional Chinese Medicine*, and *The Stories of Chinese Herbal Medicine*, etc.

It shall be noted that the efficacy and safety of some prescriptions mentioned in this book have not been validated by evidence-based medicine. Moreover, it is reported that some herbal medicines can cause irreversible damage to the human kidney and liver. As Chinese tales about Shennong tasting all kinds of herbs and Taoist magical remedies for bone injuries are unsubstantiated, those stories about Chinese herbal medicine are also unsubstantiated in this book. Therefore, it does not serve as a guide to disease prevention and treatment, and readers should consult medical professionals about specific diseases.

Due to the limited knowledge of the editors, errors might have been made in this book, and criticisms and corrections from readers are sincerely welcomed.

目　录

 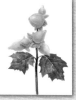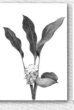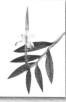

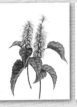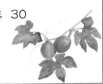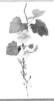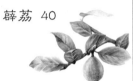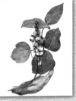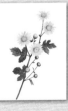

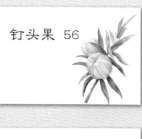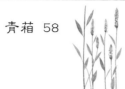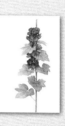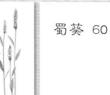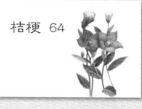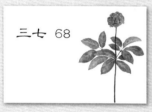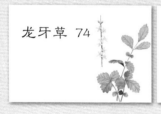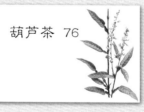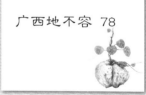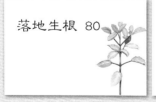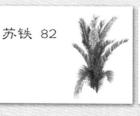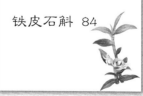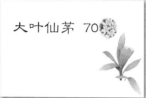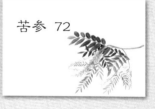

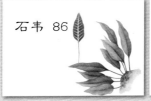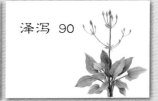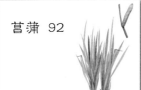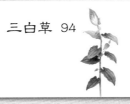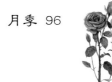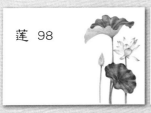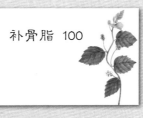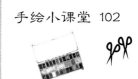

CONTENTS

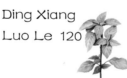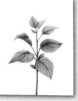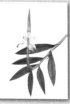

Huo Xiang 130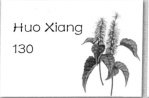

Ning Meng Cao 132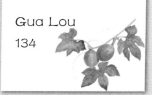

Gua Lou 134

Tian Men Dong 136

He Shou Wu 138

Fu Fang Teng 140

Shan Qian Niu 142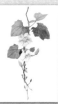

Bi Li 144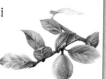

Ge 146

Hua Nan Ren Dong 148

Shui Fei Ji 150

Yi Mu Cao 152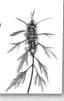

Wen Shu Lan 154

Da Che Qian 156

Ye Ju 158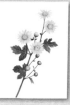

Ding Tou Guo 160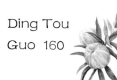

Qing Xiang 162

Shu Kui 164

Wu Yue Ai 166

Jie Geng 168

Chang Chun Hua 170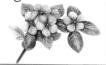

San Qi 172

Da Ye Xian Mao 174

Ku Shen 176

Long Ya Cao 178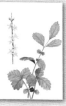

Hu Lu Cha 180

Guangxi Di Bu Rong 182

Luo Di Sheng Gen 184

Su Tie 186

Tie Pi Shi Hu 188

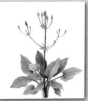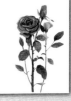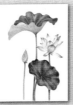

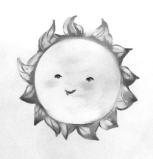

嘿，朋友们！欢迎来到草本药物园区，
你准备好认识它们了吗？

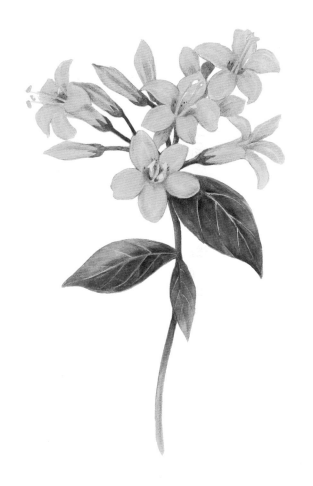

gōu wěn
钩吻

古时候的断肠草，小朋友们知多少?

李时珍在《本草纲目》中提到的"断肠草"指的是钩吻。钩吻的毒素有显著的镇痛和加强催眠的作用。

在古代，人们通常把服用以后对人体胃肠道产生强烈中毒反应的草药叫作"断肠草"，毛茛科的乌头、瑞香科的狼毒、大戟科的大戟等，都是因为具有明显的毒性而有"断肠草"之称。人一旦误食了这些"断肠草"就有可能会死亡。

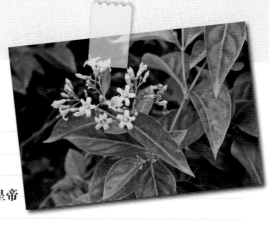

别名：断肠草、大茶药、胡蔓藤
拉丁学名：*Gelsemium elegans* Benth.

　　　　断肠草与乾隆皇帝

　　清朝年间，乾隆皇帝微服私访来到镇江。在一家客店投宿后，乾隆皇帝感到身上奇痒，便到一家草药铺买药。

　　"恕小生深夜打扰，求先生配点草药。"敲开门后，年轻儒雅的乾隆皇帝像一个富家公子一样上前行礼。

　　"客官请坐，反正我还未就寝。"一个中年郎中给他开了门。

　　乾隆皇帝将自己的病症告诉了这位郎中。郎中认真地检查后，告诉乾隆皇帝说："你患的是一种叫'疥癣'的皮肤病，能治，但需要遵医嘱。用药后不能用手直接抓挠，药更不能入口，因为此草药有剧毒。"

　　"先生能告诉我此草药的名字吗？"乾隆皇帝好奇地问。

　　"它叫'断肠草'。相传当年神农尝百草时，遇到了一种叶片相对而生的藤子，开着淡黄色小花。他摘了几片嫩叶放到口中品尝，刚嚼碎咽下，就毒性大发，肠子断成了一小段一小段的。这种藤子就被人们称为'断肠草'。"郎中回答道。

　　不久之后，乾隆皇帝的病被治愈了。他重赏了这位郎中，又挥笔为这位郎中的草药铺写下了"神农百草堂"几个大字。这个草药铺因此而名扬四海。

猜一猜

　　一行书信千行泪。（打一植物名）

（谜底：相思豆）

3

bì má

蓖麻

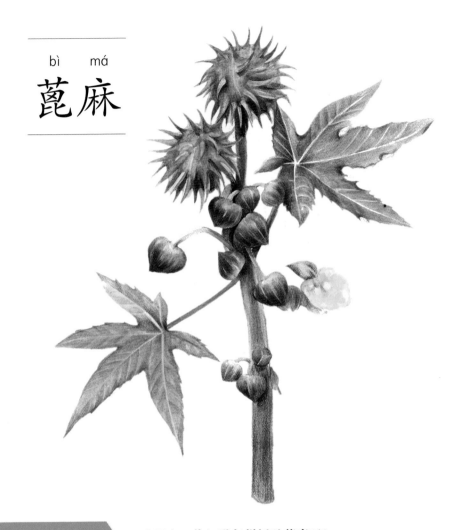

小朋友，你知道怎样播种蓖麻吗?

　　在播种前，把蓖麻种子浸泡在 40~50℃的温水中 24 小时后捞出，埋在湿润的沙子里。蓖麻种子发芽一般需要 5~7 天，发芽后就可以立即播种。

　　放置了一段时间的蓖麻种子可用 40~50℃的温水浸泡 48 小时，使种子硬壳变软，籽粒吸足水分，以加快种子的发芽速度。等到一部分蓖麻种子露芽的时候，就可以播种了。

别名：大麻子、老麻子、草麻
拉丁学名：*Ricinus communis* L.

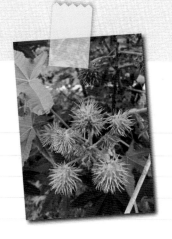

约拿和蓖麻

　　在耶罗波安二世的时代，亚述国的以色列人得到上帝的祝福和教导，却不愿意侍奉上帝。因此，上帝派了一位叫约拿的先知去警告他们：因为他们的罪恶，亚述国的尼尼微城将在 40 天内被毁灭。

　　尼尼微人收到警告后开始向上帝祷告。上帝垂听到了他们的祷告，决定不再毁灭尼尼微城。

　　约拿却不同意，还因此生闷气不理会上帝。他在一个可以俯瞰全城的地方搭了一个小棚子，观察这座城市。然而，什么事也没有发生，只有热辣辣的太阳照着他。

　　上帝栽了一棵蓖麻给约拿乘凉，这下约拿感觉凉快多了。

　　第二天，那棵蓖麻却枯萎了，原来是上帝打发了一条虫子来咬蓖麻的根。为他遮阳的蓖麻死了，而邪恶的尼尼微城却还安然无恙，这让约拿感到愤怒。

　　于是，上帝警告约拿说："这棵蓖麻不是你栽种的，也不是你培养的，你都那么爱惜。尼尼微城中的所有百姓和城里的草木，我怎能不爱惜呢？"

　　约拿听后终于明白了上帝的一番苦心。

猜一猜

　　皮儿薄，壳儿脆，四姐妹，隔墙睡，从小到大背靠背，裹着一层疙瘩被。（打一植物名）

（麻蓖：底谜）

jì yīng sù
蓟罂粟

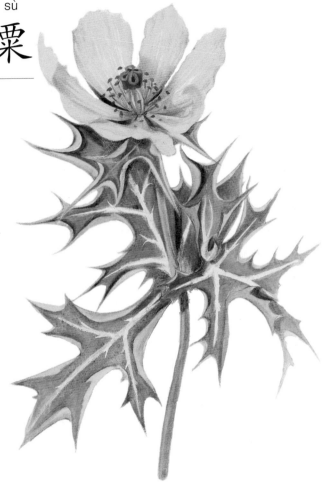

蓟罂粟把种子藏在哪儿?

　　每到夏末,蓟罂粟的果实就成熟了。采下果实,晒干,压破,除去果壳,就能取出种子了。

　　蓟罂粟的种子有毒,千万不要误食,否则会引起腹泻。

別名：刺罂粟、老鼠簕
拉丁学名：*Argemone mexicana* L.

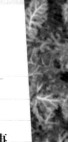

　　蓟罂粟的故事

在希腊神话中，得墨忒耳是掌管丰收和农业的女神，也是神母。得墨忒耳和统治宇宙的至高无上的主神——宙斯生了一个可爱的女儿普西芬尼。

由于得墨忒耳主管农业有方，世界上总是气候温暖，五谷丰登。

有一天，普西芬尼采花时，土地突然裂开，统治冥界的冥帝哈得斯跳出来把她劫走，将她强娶为自己的皇后。得知哈得斯抢走普西芬尼后，得墨忒耳极为痛苦，便用蓟罂粟的汁液减轻自己的痛苦和悲伤。

失去女儿的得墨忒耳再也无心管理农事。于是，大地荒芜，人类面临死亡的威胁，大神们吃不到贡物，众神之王宙斯命令哈得斯把普西芬尼送回。可是，哈得斯却强迫普西芬尼吃了一粒冥界的石榴籽，使她不能完全脱离冥界。普西芬尼每年只有 1/4 的时间能回到地上同母亲生活在一起，其余时间则住在冥界。

当普西芬尼回到地上时，得墨忒耳就会很高兴，于是春暖花开，万物开始生长；而当普西芬尼回到冥界时，得墨忒耳又被哀愁所笼罩，于是万物又开始凋零，从而导致了一年四季变化的现象。

　　中草药没有毒副作用吗？

"中草药是天然药物，没有毒副作用。"虽然类似说法在民间很流行，但是科研人员研究发现，许多中草药具有毒副作用，甚至具有很强的毒性。一些中医经典古籍记载"无毒"的中草药被发现能导致肾衰竭、癌症、胸腺萎缩、重金属中毒、畸胎等。因此，小朋友们千万不要轻信民间流传的偏方、验方，不要随便采用中药方剂，或服用中药补药和中药保健品。

商陆

shāng　lù

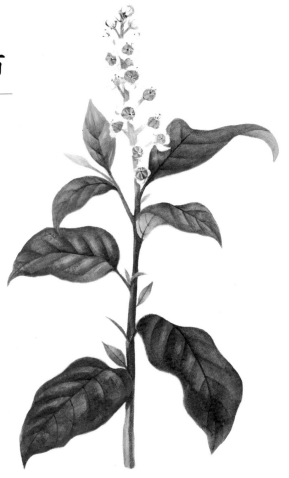

趣味小知识　　　　**商陆也能做胭脂？**

　　商陆还有一个名字叫"胭脂草"，商陆扁圆形的浆果成熟时呈深红紫色或黑色，像是微缩的葡萄。民间常把它当作胭脂涂在女孩子的额角，所以商陆也被人们称为"胭脂草"。古人云：胭脂草，女儿心。

　　商陆的果实颜色鲜艳且多汁，十分诱人，但是却有毒，小朋友们千万不能误食它。

别名：山萝卜、见肿消、夜呼
拉丁学名：*Phytolacca acinosa* Roxb.

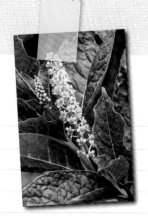

　　商陆名字的故事

　　唐玄宗开元年间，南山边上有一个道湾村，村里有一个江湖郎中名叫史夫，他跟人学了点医术，加上他那三寸不烂之舌，就自称"神医"了。

　　后来，周边的村民不再向他求医。于是他将药箱一背，写有"济世活佛、妙手回春"的幡子一举，大摇大摆地去别的地方行医了。

　　史夫来到一处漫山遍野都是坟墓的荒山野岭。一个樵夫挑着柴从山上下来，由于走得急，不小心撞到史夫，一下将史夫撞晕了过去。

　　樵夫以为史夫被他撞死了，吓得一溜烟逃跑了。

　　史夫醒来时，已经是日落西山了。他隐约听到一阵阵哭声从坟墓旁边长得非常旺盛的草里传出来。他便把草扒开，挖出一个倒圆锥形的肉质植物。因其形似萝卜，又有似人参一样的根，史夫以为自己挖了棵人参，立即一口咬下去，随后他恶心呕吐、腹痛腹泻不止，便哭着去找大夫。大夫了解情况后，翻阅医书，给史夫解了毒。

　　从此，史夫努力学习医术，再也不敢胡乱给人看病了。而那天他挖到的"人参"，因为他当时隐约听到哭声，所以史夫把它叫作"夜呼"。

猜一猜

　　三十除以五。（打一植物名）

（谜底：商陆。我国古代算式上往往以算筹中的横杆表示六，即用六根算子表示六。）

yè gān

射干

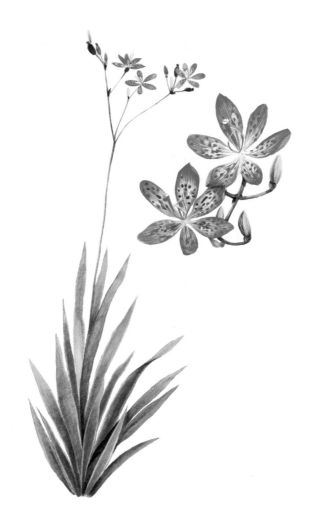

趣味小知识 ● **射干和鸢尾长得很像，如何区分它们呢？**

　　1. 射干：（1）干燥根茎是不规则的结节状；（2）表面有黄褐色或黑褐色斑点；（3）味苦。

　　2. 鸢尾：（1）干燥根茎是扁圆柱形；（2）表面呈灰棕色；（3）味苦略带辛味。

别名：野萱花、交剪草、扁竹

拉丁学名：*Belamcanda chinensis* Redouté

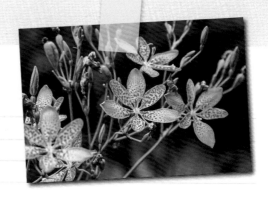

　　射干的故事

很久以前，有个樵夫住在猫儿山脚下，以砍柴为生。他需要照顾双目失明的老母亲，他们的生活过得很艰难。

有一年夏天，樵夫感冒了，咽喉疼痛，好几天没有上山砍柴。因为没钱，他只能从邻居家借来一碗米煮粥给老母亲吃。

老母亲吃完后，樵夫便拖着虚弱的身子上山砍柴。由于身体虚弱，加上没有吃东西，樵夫晕倒在了溪流边。

樵夫醒来时，发现自己躺在万花丛中，旁边有很多像蝴蝶一样漂亮的花。由于非常饥饿，樵夫忍不住吃了一棵这种带花的植物。这种植物刚入口时味道苦涩，但过后有一种甜甜的味道，嗓子还有清凉感。没过多久，樵夫的嗓子好了很多，精神也比之前要好。

这时，一位美丽善良的仙子来到樵夫的身边，告诉他这种花叫作"射干"，能治疗咽喉疼痛。

樵夫担心家中的老母亲，道谢后便急着赶回家。仙子被他的孝心感动了，送给他很多射干的种子，并告诉他怎么种植这种草药。

樵夫回到家后按照仙子教的方法，在屋子附近种了很多的这种草药，并且毫无保留地教会了乡亲们怎么种植这种草药。

从此，樵夫和乡亲们靠种植这种草药过上了衣食无忧的生活。

猜一猜

花落云飞蜓展翼。（打一中药名）

（谜底：射干）

11

rǔ　qié

乳茄

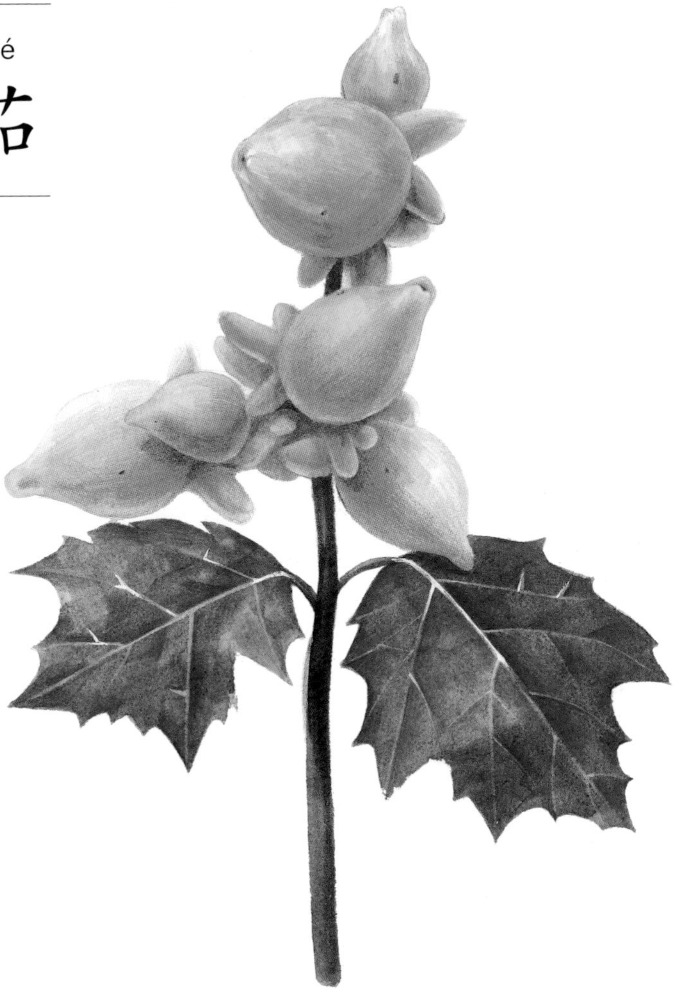

趣味小知识　　**有毒的黄金果——乳茄**

　　乳茄是盆景花卉中的新宠，因其果实形状酷似乳房而得名。其果实经久不变色、不干缩，金光灿灿，象征财运高照、五代同堂、吉祥如意，又有五子登科之意，故被用作年花。但是乳茄有毒，不可随便生食，否则会对身体造成伤害。

别名：五指茄、五角丁茄、五子登科
拉丁学名：*Solanum mammosum* L.

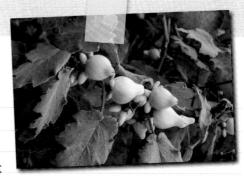

五角丁茄的故事

在神秘的古代，美丽的美洲有一个印第安人居住的村庄。村庄里有一对兄弟，弟弟从小体弱，哥哥便一心一意地照顾弟弟。哥哥每天都到森林打猎，弟弟就在村庄附近采摘野果。

这天，哥哥由于追赶猎物过急，不小心滚落壕沟。他在滚落中扭伤了脚，还撞到了一棵大树，昏了过去。因森林里很潮湿，哥哥身上的伤口感染了。

弟弟靠在门边等哥哥，等着等着就睡着了。梦里，一位树仙子把哥哥的情况告诉了弟弟。弟弟吓得哭了，赶紧询问树仙子如何才能找到哥哥。树仙子给弟弟指引了一条小路，并告诉弟弟："我身边长有一丛茎有短柔毛及扁刺，结着有五个角状凸起的金色肚形果实的直立的草。你把小金果采回家后晒干，敷在伤口上，可以治疗你哥哥身上的痈肿。"

弟弟醒来后，立刻按照梦里树仙子指引的路找到哥哥并把他搀扶回家。他还在大树附近找到树仙子所说的小金果，采摘了一些带回家，按树仙子的教导为哥哥疗伤，不久哥哥就痊愈了。

之后，兄弟俩来到树下对树仙子表示敬意和感激，并给丁点大的小金果起名"五角丁茄"。

五个儿子中状元。（打一植物名）

（谜底：五子登科）

yáng jīn huā

洋金花

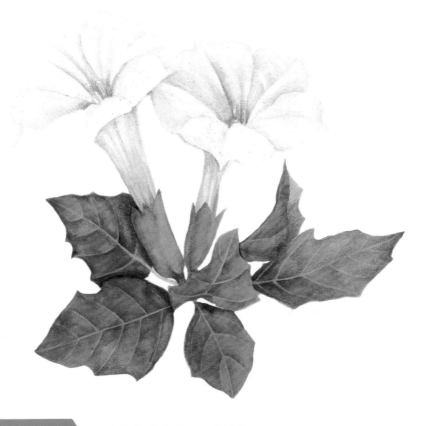

趣味小知识 ▶ **古老的麻醉剂——麻沸散**

　　相传，我国名医华佗早在公元 200 年左右，就曾用麻沸散作为麻醉剂为患者施行刮骨、剖腹术（此传说明显违背科学常识，缺乏考古证据佐证）。麻沸散就是用洋金花制成的中药麻醉剂。

别名：白花曼陀罗、闹羊花、臭麻子花
拉丁学名：*Datura metel* L.

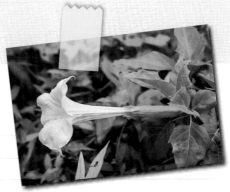

最早的麻醉剂——麻沸散

相传，有一天，华佗行医时碰到一位奇怪的患者：患者牙关紧闭，口吐白沫，手攥拳，躺在地上不动弹。华佗上前看他的神态，按他的脉搏，摸他的额头，发现一切都正常。华佗就问患者家人，患者有过什么疾病，患者的家人说："他身体非常健壮，什么疾病都没有，就是今天误吃了几朵臭麻子花（即洋金花），才出现这些症状。"

华佗连忙让他们找些臭麻子花来看看。患者的家人把一棵连花带果的臭麻子花送到华佗面前，华佗接过臭麻子花闻了闻，看了看，又摘了一朵花放在嘴里尝了尝，顿时觉得头晕目眩，满嘴发麻。

华佗用清凉解毒的办法治愈了这位患者。临走时，他什么也没要，只要了一捆连花带果的臭麻子花。

从那天起，华佗开始用臭麻子花进行试验，他先尝叶，后尝花，最后尝果和根。试验结果表明，臭麻子果的麻醉效果很好。华佗到处走访了许多医生，收集了一些有麻醉作用的药物，经过多次不同配方的炮制，终于研制出了麻醉药。他把热酒加入麻醉药中，结果麻醉效果更好。

华佗给配好的麻醉药方起了一个名字——麻沸散。

秋色从西来。（打一植物名）

（谜底：洋金花）

dīng xiāng luó lè

丁香罗勒

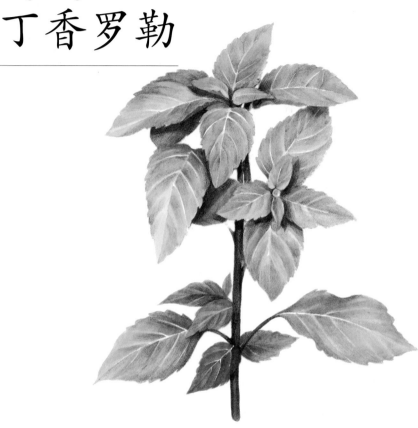

趣味小知识 ▶ **罗勒精油用处大**

1. 罗勒精油对呼吸系统有帮助，可治疗感冒、咳嗽，有助于减轻气喘、支气管炎、鼻腔黏膜炎等症状，还可以治疗消化不良。

2. 罗勒精油可以缓解沮丧，振作精神，使人感觉敏锐；有镇静作用，缓解歇斯底里的症状表现；还能减轻头痛。

3. 罗勒精油可紧实肌肤，平衡油脂分泌；罗勒精油对敏感性皮肤略具刺激性。

别名：臭草
拉丁学名：*Ocimum gratissimum* L.

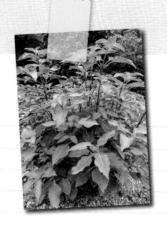

丁香罗勒的传说

很久以前，一个美丽的女孩爱上了一个英俊的男孩，男孩家境贫寒。镇上住着一个富豪，他一直钟情于女孩，并且曾经多次上门说亲，但都遭到女孩的拒绝。而女孩的家人一心想让女孩嫁给富豪，好让他们的生活得到改善。

女孩的两个哥哥非常痛恨那个男孩，认为是男孩破坏了他们过上好日子的美梦。于是两个哥哥多次设下陷阱栽赃陷害男孩，想让女孩放弃跟男孩在一起的想法。但是两个哥哥的阴谋每次都被识破，女孩最后还是跟男孩在一起了，而且他们的感情越来越牢固。

为了让两个哥哥死心，女孩打算跟男孩在七夕那天定亲。两个哥哥知道这个消息后几乎要崩溃，他们决定杀死男孩。

终于有一天，女孩的两个哥哥把男孩骗到荒郊野外，并将其杀害。女孩得知此事后非常伤心，整整哭了七天七夜，最后她在男孩被杀害的地方种了一株罗勒。

第二年，罗勒便散发出一股丁香的芬芳。此后，这种植物就有一股醉人的丁香的香气，因此而得名"丁香罗勒"。

猜一猜

四棱茎，气芳香，紫花绿叶，驱蚊好。（打一植物名）

（谜底：丁香罗勒）

zǐ sū
紫苏

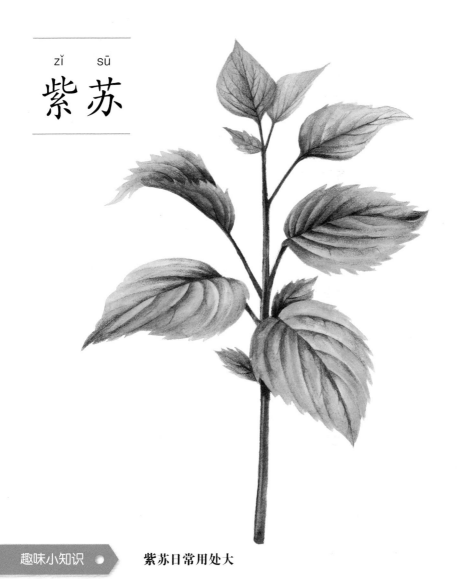

紫苏日常用处大

　　紫苏在我们日常生活中的用处可大了。它可以用来作香料和配菜，也可以用来解虾、蟹等海鲜的毒性。另外它还可以治疗感冒，夏季如果得了风寒感冒、恶寒发热、咳嗽、气喘、胸腹胀满等，可以喝用紫苏嫩叶煮的汤或生吃紫苏嫩叶，很有效哦。

别名：赤苏、红苏、红紫苏

拉丁学名：*Perilla frutescens* Britt.

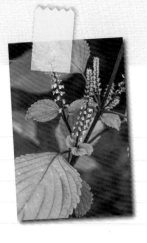

　　　紫苏的传说

　　相传，在九月九日重阳节这一天，华佗带着徒弟去镇上。途中，忽见一只水獭逮住了一条大鱼，并把大鱼连鳞带骨都吞进了肚里。把大鱼全都吃完后，水獭撑得难受极了，在岸边翻滚折腾。后来，只见水獭爬到岸边一块紫草地旁，吃了些紫草叶，又爬了几圈，不一会儿它便舒坦自如地游走了。

　　到了镇上，师徒俩在一个酒铺里饮酒。旁边几个少年在比赛吃螃蟹。华佗想，螃蟹性寒，吃多了会生病，便上前好言相劝。那伙少年哪听得进华佗的良言！其中一个少年还讽刺说："老头儿，你是不是眼馋了，我掰一块给你尝尝。"

　　华佗叹息一声，只好坐下来喝自己的酒。

　　哪知过了一个时辰，那伙少年突然都喊肚子疼。有的疼得额上冒汗珠，喊爹喊娘地直叫，有的捧着肚子在地上翻滚。

　　坐在旁边的华佗就叫徒弟在这酒铺外的洼地里采些紫草叶给他们吃，少年们服用后不久肚子就不疼了。他们再三向华佗表示感谢，回家后到处向人讲华佗医术如何高明。

　　因为这种药草是紫色的，吃后很舒服，所以华佗给它取名"紫舒"。后来因为音近，人们把它叫作"紫苏"。

猜一猜 ●

　　从来没赢过。（打一植物名）

（谜底：紫苏，即"总输"，谐音。）

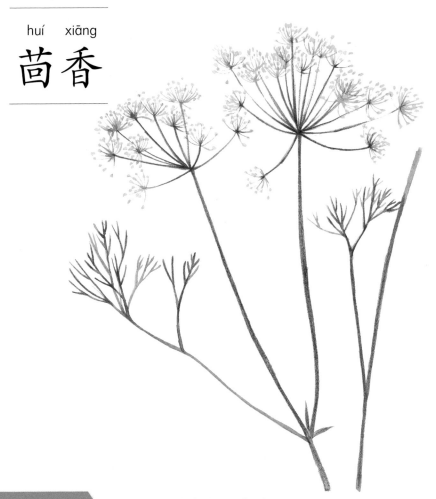

huí xiāng
茴香

茴香和孜然是同一种东西吗?

很多读者在日常生活中都见过孜然粉和茴香,那么它们是不是同一种东西呢?相信很多读者都不知道,下面,我们来看看它们的区别吧。

它们虽然都是香辛料,形状差不多,但味道不一样。且茴香个头稍大,颗粒有点胖,颜色发绿;孜然稍细长,颜色发黄。读者朋友,你会区分它们了吗?

别名：小·茴香、土茴香
拉丁学名：*Foeniculum vulgare* Mill.

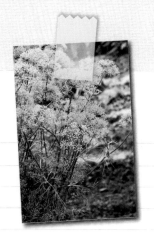

　　富商疝气和小茴香的故事

　　清朝末年，一位名叫米哈伊洛夫的俄罗斯富商来到中国。早就听说乾隆皇帝流连江南美景的他，也想去领略江南的风光。有一天，他也下江南，乘船游览杭州西湖。正当他尽情欣赏秀丽风光之时，突然疝气发作，痛得他捧腹大叫，还在地上打滚。随行的俄罗斯医生都慌了，焦急地看着米哈伊洛夫被病痛折磨，却束手无策。正在万分紧急的时候，船夫看见此情况，赶紧推荐了一位老中医给他们。

　　在这个紧要关头，俄罗斯医生也只好放手，让老中医来施展医术。只见老中医不慌不忙地取出中药小茴香一两，研成粗末，让米哈伊洛夫用二两浙江绍兴黄酒送服。大约过了20分钟，米哈伊洛夫的疝痛果然奇迹般地减轻并很快消失了。随行的俄罗斯医生都十分惊讶，这小小的种粒居然能治这种突发的怪病，都纷纷向老中医寻求秘方。老中医毫不吝啬地告诉他们：是小茴香的种子治好了米哈伊洛夫的病。

　　得知自己的疼痛是被小茴香治好的，米哈伊洛夫大呼神奇，同时也对中医的神奇深感敬佩，此事一时被传为佳话。

猜一猜

　　半部春秋反复念。（打一中药名）

（谜底：茴香）

21

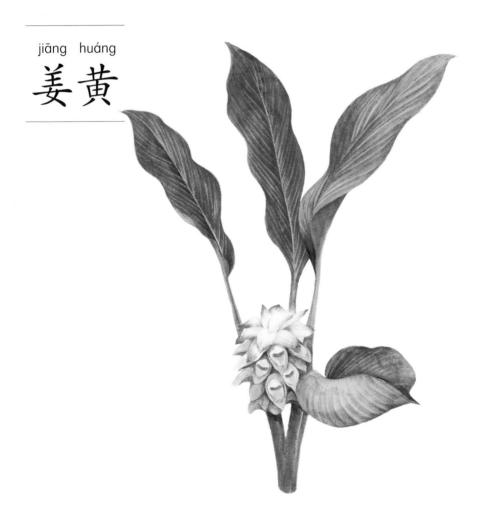

jiāng huáng

姜黄

姜黄除了做药还有什么用处呢?

　　下面我们一起来看看姜黄在日常生活中还有什么用处吧。姜黄属于生姜植物家族，经常被用作香料添加到食物中。姜黄粉是最常见的形式，它是姜黄根茎经过煮熟干燥后碾成的橘黄色粉末。姜黄粉可作为食品添加剂，是咖喱粉中的重要成分。此外，制作泡菜等食品也需要使用姜黄。

别名：宝鼎香、黄姜、郁金
拉丁学名：*Curcuma longa* L.

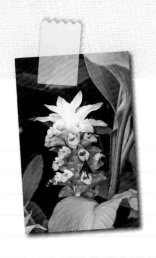

姜黄的故事

　　相传，在很早以前，汉江及天河流域连续三年遭遇大旱，农作物颗粒无收。就连在天河口集镇上开饭馆的老板也外出逃荒，只留下烧火的伙夫在店内看门。这伙夫平时干活勤奋，待人厚道，周围的人称他"火头军"。

　　一天傍晚，店里来了一个瘸腿的讨饭老头儿，"火头军"把仅有的一碗红薯糊汤给他吃了。"火头军"询问老头儿家在何处，老头儿回答说住天河山里头。话音刚落，老头儿就不见了。

　　"火头军"对老头儿放心不下，第二天就上山寻找他。到了中午，"火头军"又累又饿，因体力不支晕倒在路旁。迷糊之中，"火头军"见一老头儿低着头在山坡上挖出一种带毛的根茎，然后放入锅内蒸煮。"火头军"再仔细看了看，原来就是昨天晚上的那个老头儿。他正要上前细问时，就惊醒了。他发现自己躺在密密麻麻的姜黄之上，顿觉有了精神，顺着茎叶向下挖出好多好多带毛的根茎。

　　"火头军"把这些根茎带回家，按照梦中那老头儿的方法蒸煮它，熟后剥皮食之，味道可口清香。周围的人吃了之后，都觉得这根茎既味美又可充饥。于是一传十，十传百，姜黄的故事很快传遍了天河沿岸。

　　一个黄妈妈，一生手段辣，老来愈厉害，小孩最怕他。（打一植物名）

（谜底：姜黄）

23

yì　zhì

益智

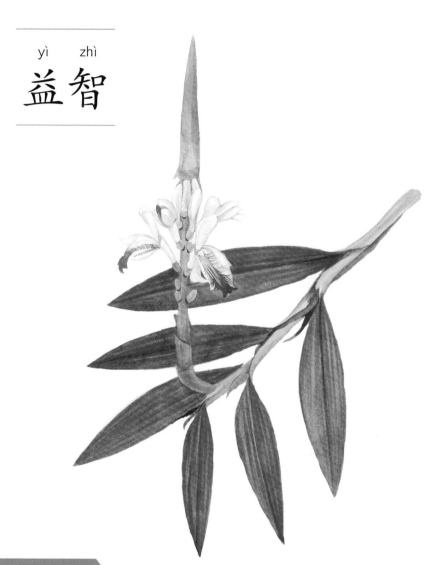

益智和姜长得很像，我们如何区分它们呢？

　　首先，从药用部位看，姜供药用的是块茎，而益智用的是果实，其果实在夏秋间变红时采收；其次，姜的块茎是不规则的，而益智的果实呈椭圆形，两端略尖，有纵向凹凸不平的凸起棱线，还有特异的香气。

别名：益智子、益智仁、摘艼子
拉丁学名：*Alpinia oxyphylla* Miq.

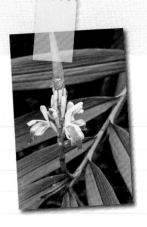

　　益智仁的传说

　　相传很久以前，有一个家财万贯的员外，年过半百才得一子，员外为其子取名叫来福。来福自小体弱多病，头长得特别大，又常流口水，而且反应迟钝，呆滞木讷，还每天尿床。一晃几年过去了，来福一直少言寡语，记性特别差，10岁了还不会数数，数到后面就忘记前面。为了给儿子治病，员外把周边的名医都请遍了，还是治不好儿子的病。

　　有一天，一个老道云游到此，听员外讲了孩子的情况后，便告诉员外说："离此地八千里的地方有一种仙果，可以治好孩子的病。"并在地上画了一幅画，画中是一棵小树，小树的叶子长得像姜叶，根部还长着几颗橄榄核状的果实，画完之后老道便走了。

　　员外决定亲自去寻找仙果，历经千辛万苦找到后，他从那棵树上摘了满满一袋果实就踏上了回家之路。

　　来福吃了员外摘回来的仙果后，变得开朗活泼、聪颖可爱，与之前相比简直判若两人。在18岁那年他去参加科举考试，结果高中状元。人们为了纪念改变来福命运的仙果，便将仙果取名为"状元果"，同时也由于它能益智、强智，使人聪明，所以又叫它"益智仁"。

猜一猜

　　使你变聪明。（打一中药名）

（谜底：益智）

25

huò xiāng

藿香

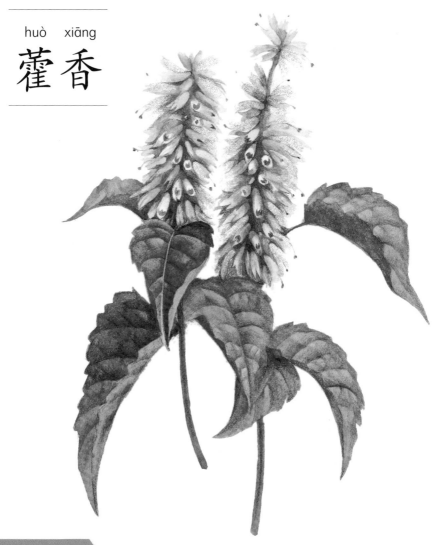

趣味小知识 ▶ **藿香除了可以用来做藿香正气水，还有很多用处呢!**

1. 园林上，藿香常成片栽植于花径、池畔和庭院。

2. 营养上，藿香是高钙、高胡萝卜素食品，全草含芳香挥发油，对多种致病性真菌有一定的抑制作用，芳香挥发油是多种中成药的原料之一。

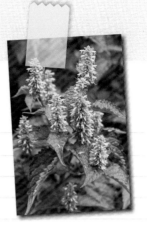

别名：合香、叶藿香、苏藿香

拉丁学名：*Agastache rugosa* O. Ktze.

　　霍香的传说

很久以前，深山里住着一户人家，家里只有哥哥和妹妹霍香两人，他们相依为命。哥哥娶亲后就从军在外，家里只剩姑嫂二人相互照顾。

有一年夏天，嫂子因劳累中暑，突然发热恶寒、头痛恶心、倦怠乏力。霍香急忙把嫂子扶到床上，并决定进深山给嫂子采治病的草药。

霍香一去就是一天，直到天黑才回来。她手里提着一小筐草药，两眼发直，一进门便扑倒在地。嫂子连忙下床扶她起来，并询问缘由，才知她在采药时，不慎被毒蛇咬伤了。嫂子一面惊叫，一面抱起霍香的右脚，准备用嘴从伤口处吸出毒汁。但霍香因怕嫂子中毒，死活不肯。等乡亲们听见嫂子的呼救将郎中找来，却为时已晚。

嫂子用霍香采来的草药治好了病，并在乡亲们的帮助下埋葬了霍香。为牢记霍香之情，嫂子便把这种有香味的草药亲切地称为"霍香"，并让大家把它种植在房前屋后、地边路旁，以便随时采用。从此霍香的名声越传越广，治好了不少中暑的病人。后来，因为是草药的缘故，人们便在"霍"字头上加了一个草字头，将"霍香"写成了"藿香"。

猜一猜

站队买东西。（打一中药名）

（谜底：藿香，即"货香"。省略。）

níng méng cǎo

柠檬草

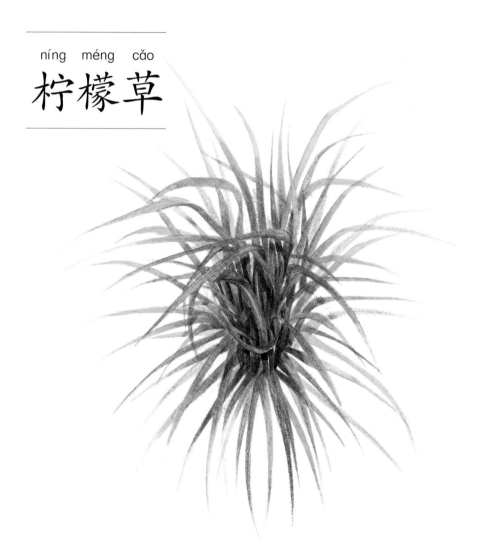

趣味小知识 ● **柠檬草精油是怎样提取的呢？**

　　提取柠檬草精油最常用的方法是水蒸气蒸馏法。具体做法是将柠檬草的花、叶、皮、根等放在蒸馏锅里，通入水蒸气，把芳香油分和水同时蒸馏出来，经冷凝器冷却后，将水油分离，分离出来的油即柠檬草精油。

别名：香茅、香麻、柠檬茅
拉丁学名：*Cymbopogon citratus*
　　　　　Stapf

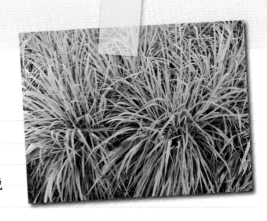

　　　　柠檬草的传说

相传，天上有一位美丽的天使，她的名字叫作雪柠，她对人间有着特殊的感情，十分向往人间。

有一天，雪柠终于来到了人间，落到了一块长满柠檬草的草坪上。她很开心，伴着柠檬草的幽香，欢快地跳起了优美的舞蹈。这时，刚好有一位英俊的王子骑着白马经过，他那蓝宝石似的眼睛一眼就看见了雪柠，王子看呆了，他对雪柠一见钟情。

回过神后，王子走到雪柠旁边向她打招呼。雪柠一回眸，也对这位王子一见钟情。之后，两人坠入爱河，过了一段让人羡慕的日子。

但是，好景不长，两人相爱的事情被主宰神界的天神知道了，他大发雷霆。因为一直以来都有一个规定：人和天使不可以相爱，若相爱就要把他们的情丝抽走，并永远冰封在玄冰森林里。

结果，王子和雪柠宁死也不愿意抽去情丝，他们央求天神让他们永远在一起。天神被他们的爱情感动了，就把他们的心和情丝化成柠檬草，而柠檬草的花语是开不了口的爱。

天神还给了柠檬草一个祝福：如果两个相恋的人拥有柠檬草就能永远在一起。

歇后语

墙上的香茅草——随风倒。

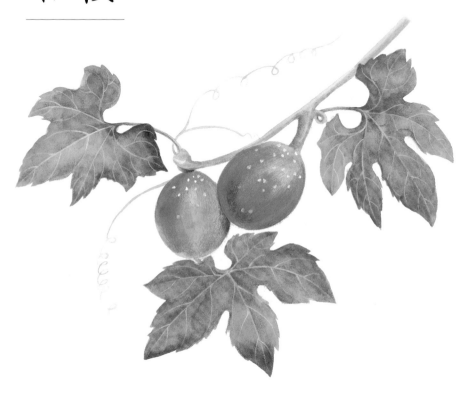

栝楼

guā lóu

天花粉是粉吗?

　　说到天花粉，或许有读者会认为它是粉末状的东西。其实，天花粉是一个中药名，是葫芦科植物栝楼的块根，名字里带有"粉"字，却没有粉的形态。

　　在明代，陈嘉谟认为：栝楼的根名为天花粉，是由于栝楼根内的花纹是天然而成的。而李时珍认为：用栝楼的根磨成的细粉洁白如雪，所以称栝楼的根为天花粉。

别名：瓜蒌、瓜楼、药瓜
拉丁学名：*Trichosanthes kirilowii*
Maxim.

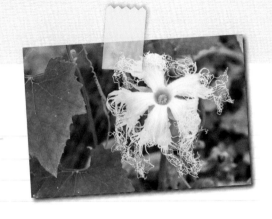

栝楼的故事

清代年间，华北山间有一个村庄，村里住着一个 15 岁的小伙子和他母亲，他们的日子过得很穷苦。

有一天夜里，小伙子梦见一个白胡子老人对他说："咱们是邻居，我就住在你家对门，没事来找老朽玩吧！"

第二天早晨，小伙子就到那里看了看，却什么也没看到。他正在那里发呆时，忽见乱草里有一缕缕从没见过的绿秧子长出来。他小心翼翼地拔净了周遭的野草，隔三岔五地还去看看，怕绿秧子被牛羊给啃了。那绿秧子长得挺旺盛，还结出一个个小绿瓜来。他不敢碰也不敢摸，像宝贝似的护着它们。

秋风凉了，那些绿瓜变得黄澄澄的，跟金瓜一样。这天夜里，小伙子又梦见了那个白胡子老人，老人笑眯眯地对他说："小伙子，你是个勤劳的好心人，待老朽太好了，明天你把那些瓜摘下来，拿到同济堂药铺卖了吧！"小伙子醒后，照着白胡子老人说的办，果然卖了不少钱。听药铺的人说，这瓜叫栝楼，根和仁都是治病的药材。

娘儿俩把那些栝楼移到自家院子里来种，没几年工夫就富裕起来了。他们还手把手地教乡亲们种栝楼，让大伙都富裕了起来。

南天门的栝楼——悬蛋。

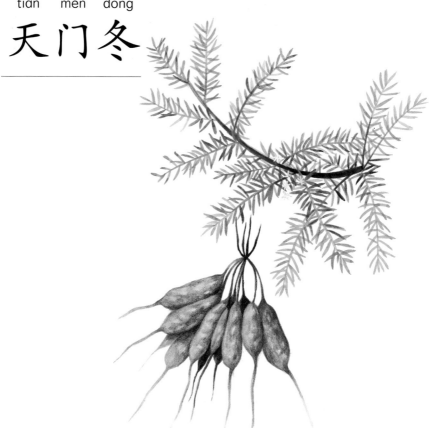

tiān mén dōng
天门冬

　　怎样种天门冬？

　　1.购买天门冬种子,于2~3月在盆内播种,放在室内,保持14~18℃的室温,要求土壤湿润、肥沃、疏松,一个月后就会长出小苗。长苗后可分株,即将茎蔓繁密的母株用刀分割开后,分别栽植在新的花盆和新的培养土中养护。

　　2.直接种新鲜的天门冬块根。天门冬的根系生长很快,每年早春,除补充新的培养土外,还需要剪去部分老根和部分攀缘老茎。

32

别名：三百棒、丝冬、老虎尾巴根
拉丁学名：*Asparagus cochinchinensis* Merr.

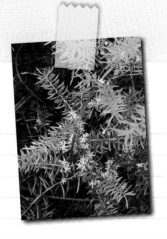

　　　　天门冬的故事

　　明代末年，爆发了大规模的农民起义，起义军的领袖名叫李自成。为了联合大将张献忠攻打明代王朝，李自成决定亲自去拜会张献忠。

　　不巧，李自成去拜访之日，张献忠的夫人正在生产，张献忠只好让他的副将出来迎接李自成。

　　李自成等了半个时辰，还不见张献忠出现，非常生气，于是一掌拍在桌子上，吼道："张献忠竟然如此怠慢于我！"

　　副将吓坏了，急忙解释道："大帅请息怒，张将军确实是因夫人生产，离不得身。大帅先尝尝这个，张将军马上就来。"

　　李自成见仆人端上一盘佐茶食品，色泽鲜亮，异香扑鼻，玉洁冰清，随口问道："这是何物？"

　　副将答道："这是天门冬蜜饯，请品尝。"

　　李自成品尝后，感觉这蜜饯味道甜美，滋润化渣，妙不可言。于是，李自成慢慢消了怒火，称赞道："果然美味。"

　　副将看到李自成消了怒气，又说道："这天门冬不仅好吃，还能滋阴润肺，清肺降火。大帅少安毋躁，张将军马上就来。"

　　又过了半个时辰，张献忠夫人顺利产下孩子后，张献忠立即赶来客厅与李自成商议攻打之事。

　　琼楼玉宇，高处不胜寒。（打一药材名）

（答案：天门冬）

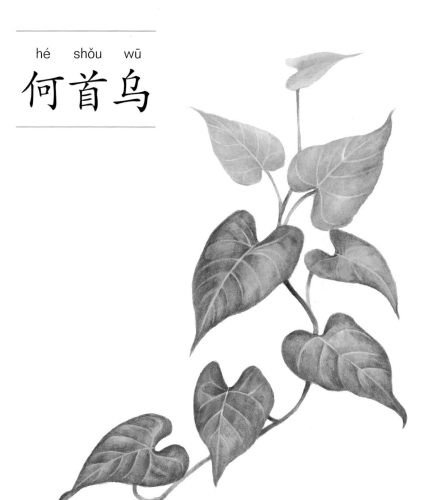

hé shǒu wū
何首乌

趣味小知识 ▶ **何首乌藤茎为何叫作夜交藤?**

　　传说到了夜里,即使相隔三尺多远,何首乌的藤茎也会互相交合,交合很长时间后又自行分开,一晚上分分合合三四次,因此,何首乌藤也叫"夜交藤"。

别名：多花蓼、紫乌藤、夜交藤
拉丁学名：*Pleuropterus multiflorus* Nakai

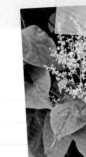

何首乌的传说

很久很久以前，地方官府常压迫老百姓去做苦役。

有一座不知名的山，山里有一个村子，村子里有一个皮肤黝黑、头发花白的可怜农夫。有一天，他不幸被官府抓去做苦役。白天，农夫被押到野外的山上辛苦劳作，到了晚上他被关进漆黑的牢房，还常常挨饿。

一天夜里，农夫饥饿难忍，他发现牢窗上有很多植物的藤茎蔓延进来，于是他便扯这种植物的茎叶来充饥。之后的每天夜里，农夫都用这种植物的茎叶来填饱肚子。

后来，农夫很幸运地得到了释放。他高兴地把牢窗外的植物连根挖出来，用衣服包好，历尽艰辛把它带回了家。农夫回到村里时，村里的人都认不出他了！原本做了几年苦役的他应该更苍老、更憔悴，可是他看起来却越发年轻了。不仅花白的头发变成了乌黑的青丝，整个人也容光焕发了。村里人都很惊诧，便问其故。农夫拿出包在衣服里的植物，说："关在牢里的时候，我天天夜里都用它来充饥。"大家都不知道这植物叫什么名字，因为农夫姓何，于是大家把这种植物命名为"何首乌"。

返老还童。（打一中药名）

（谜底：何首乌）

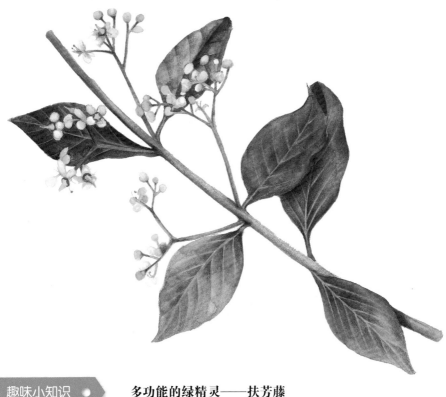

fú fāng téng
扶芳藤

　　　　多功能的绿精灵——扶芳藤

　　扶芳藤可铺地、绕树，也可爬墙。它不仅是提高绿化覆盖率的攀缘植物，也是立体绿化的好材料。它不但生长迅速、萌发力强、生态功能强、极耐修剪，还养护简单，不需要过多的水分。

　　扶芳藤能吸收二氧化硫、三氧化硫、氯气、氟化氢、二氧化氮等有害气体，可作为空气污染严重工矿区的环境绿化树种。

别名：换骨筋、爬藤、爬行卫矛
拉丁学名：*Euonymus fortunei* Hand.
-Mazz.

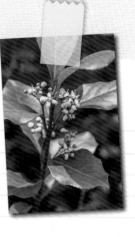

扶芳藤的故事

很久以前，有一户农家，家里很穷，还养着四个孩子，仅仅靠耕种田地根本不足以养活家里那么多口人。因此，父亲就决定上山，想挖些珍贵的药材换钱来补贴家用。

刚开始，父亲还是很容易挖到像灵芝这类的珍贵药材。后来，村里的人得知挖药材可以换钱后，都上山去挖药材赚钱。渐渐地父亲就很难挖到药材了。

有一次上山挖药，父亲空手而归。回到家看着瘦弱的孩子，父亲心里十分难受。于是，晚上他跟孩子的母亲商量，决定到很远的深山里找找，看能否找到珍贵药材。

第二天天刚蒙蒙亮，父亲就带着干粮出门了。他走了很久很久，来到了深山里头，发现陡峭的山崖边上有一棵很大很珍贵的药材。于是他就往上爬，不料一失足摔了下来，跌伤了腿。他无法行走，于是随手抓起身边的植物捣碎敷在腿上。过了很久，感觉腿不怎么痛了，父亲慢慢站起来，缓缓行走回家。

之后，父亲便把这植物挖回家种植，每次去深山挖药时都随身带一些，以预防摔伤。后来人们就知道了这种植物可用来医治跌打损伤，所以有的地方又把它叫作"换骨筋"。

猜一猜

小小植物爱攀缘，一攀攀到房顶上。
朵朵小花聚成伞，冬天更赛爬山虎。（打一植物名）

（谜底：扶芳藤）

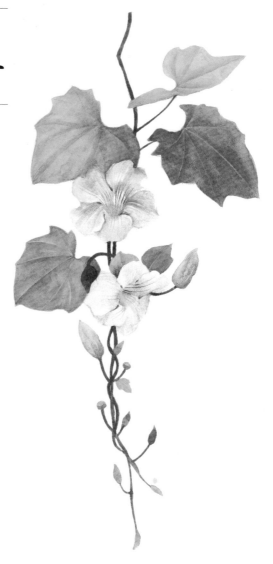

山牵牛

shān qiān niú

你知道山牵牛为什么又叫孟加拉右旋藤吗?

山牵牛原产于孟加拉国,株高 7 米以上,有很强的攀爬性,藤蔓长 20 米以上。因为它的藤蔓总是右旋攀爬,所以又有"孟加拉右旋藤"之称。

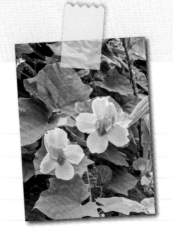

别名：大花山牵牛、大花老鸦嘴、
　　　孟加拉右旋藤
拉丁学名：*Thunbergia grandiflora* Roxb.

　　　山牵牛的故事

　　从前，在一个村子里，有一个很自傲的人，他喜欢跑进山里去抓蛇，由于从来没有失过手，因此自称是村里的"蛇老大"。"蛇老大"经常向村里其他人夸自己很了不起，还常常看不起其他抓蛇的人。

　　最近，村里经常丢失牲口，像鸡、羊等。一开始人们觉得很奇怪，后来大家偷偷观察，发现原来是有一条蛇来偷吃他们的牲口。人们几次想抓住它，但是这条蛇很聪明，几次都逃过村里人的抓捕。村里人实在没有办法，便去请"蛇老大"。"蛇老大"扬扬得意地来到蛇穴处，设下关卡想引蛇出洞。不料那条蛇好像跟他有仇似的，不但没被抓着，反而咬了他一口，他痛得不停地在地上打滚。正巧，这一幕被村里另一个抓蛇的小伙子看到，小伙子赶紧抓起一些形似喇叭的植物捣碎敷在"蛇老大"的伤口上，渐渐地，"蛇老大"的伤口就不疼了。

　　后来，小伙子帮村里人抓住了这条蛇，还告诉大家，这种植物可以治疗蛇咬伤。因为它跟牵牛花长得很像，又生长在山里，所以人们把它叫作"山牵牛"。

　　最爱爬篱笆，朵朵开像大喇叭。（打一植物名）

（谜底：山牵牛）

39

bì lì

薜荔

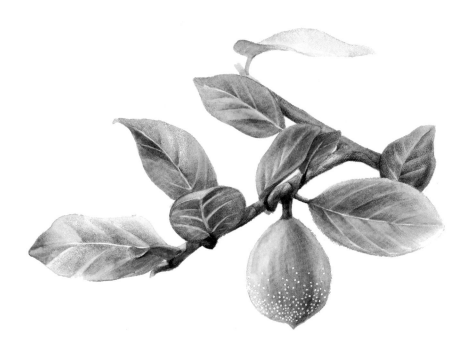

白凉粉的原料——薜荔

  相信小朋友们都吃过白凉粉吧，薜荔是制作白凉粉的原料。将薜荔果实的籽用布袋装着放在适量凉开水中，不断揉搓挤捏，把籽中的胶质挤出来。然后加入适量凝固剂，凝固后，晶莹剔透的白凉粉就制作好了。在炎热的夏天，吃上一口冰镇的白凉粉，那是多么美好的一件事啊！

别名：凉粉子、木莲、凉粉果
拉丁学名：*Ficus pumila* L.

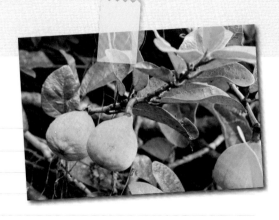

　　薜荔的故事

　　从前，在美丽的台湾有一个可爱的女孩，父母给她取名"爱玉"。爱玉的家里非常贫穷，养不起她，父母便把幼小的爱玉送去富人家里干活。

　　有一天，爱玉帮富人家送东西到村里，经过一条清澈的小河边时，她那饿极了的小肚子"咕噜噜"地叫起来。这时，她发现河面上漂来一个黄澄澄的东西，就顺手捞起这块柔软透明的黄色晶体。爱玉仔细观察了一阵，最后还是决定把这块看起来能填饱肚子的东西吃掉。品尝过后，爱玉发现这块黄色晶体竟然如此甘甜可口。

　　爱玉仔细地观察小河的周围，想知道这美味的食物到底是从哪里漂来的。在河边，她发现一株木莲藤的果实掉落河水后，在水里凝结而成一个黄澄澄的透明晶体，就像她刚才捞起来吃的那种食物。

　　爱玉非常高兴，她把这种黄澄澄的晶体带回村子，把她在小河边捞起黄色晶体并吃掉的经过告诉村里的人。村里的人知道之后也跑去河边吃这种晶体。从此，这种食物被叫作"爱玉"。

　　后来，人们才知道这种果实是凉粉果，在水里凝结成的透明晶体叫"凉粉"，而结这种果实的植物叫"薜荔"。

　　槛前衰草紧相连。（打一植物名）

（谜底：木槿）

gě

葛

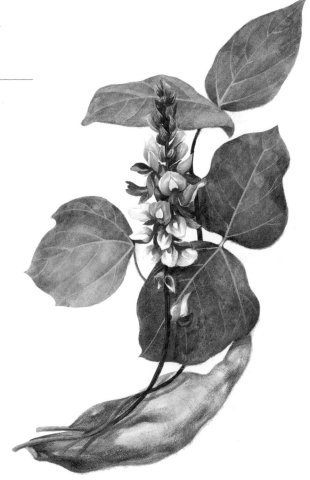

如何挑选葛根?

1. 看颜色。真葛根外表呈白色或淡棕色，有时可见残存的棕色外皮；假葛根表面呈棕褐色，具不规则的细裂纹、纵皱和不明显的皮孔样突起。

2. 闻气味。真葛根闻之无味，口尝味微甜；假葛根闻之亦气微，但口尝味微苦。

别名：野葛、葛藤
拉丁学名：*Pueraria montana* var. *lobata*

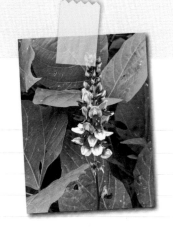

　　葛的故事

　　相传，盛唐年间，在某个山脚下住着一对夫妻，男的名字叫付郎，女的名字叫畲女，付郎专心读书，畲女辛勤耕作。经过十年寒窗苦读，付郎终于高中进士，这本来是一件非常令人高兴的事情，付郎却烦恼满怀。因为在长安城里，付郎看到富人家的女子个个艳若牡丹，丰盈美丽。想想自己的妻子因长年劳作，瘦弱不堪，于是想要休掉畲女。他托乡人带信回家，畲女拆开信，只见两句诗："缘似落花如流水，驿道春风是牡丹。"畲女明白付郎要将自己抛弃，非常伤心，终日以泪洗面，吃不下饭，容颜变得更加憔悴。

　　山神得知后，怜爱善良苦命的畲女，便在梦中指引畲女每日到山上挖食葛根。不久，畲女竟脱胎换骨，变得丰盈美丽，光彩照人。

　　乡人走后，付郎思来想去：同甘共苦多年的妻子，怎能抛弃？！于是他快马加鞭，赶回故里，发现妻子变得异常美丽，不由得大喜过望，夫妻团圆，共享荣华。从此畲族女子便有了吃食葛根的习俗，而且个个胸臀丰满、体态苗条、肤色白皙。

　　老葛家的独生子。（打一药材名）

（谜底：葛根）

43

huá nán rěn dōng

华南忍冬

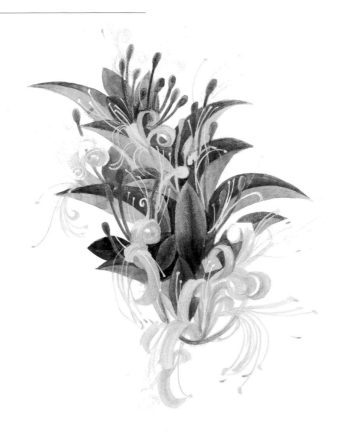

趣味小知识 ▶ **华南忍冬还有什么有趣的名字？**

　　华南忍冬，三月开花，微香，蒂带红色，花初开色白，经一两日则色黄，所以又名"金银花"。又因为一蒂二花，两朵花的花蕊匀探在外，成双成对，形影不离，犹如雄雌相伴，又似鸳鸯对舞，故有"鸳鸯藤"之称。

44

别名：大金银花、山金银花、土银花
拉丁学名：*Lonicera confusa* DC.

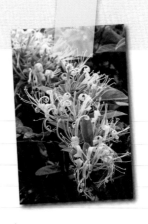

草药小故事　　**金银花的传说**

一千五百年前，在中州大地一个叫黄池的地方，居住着一位姓黄的神医。他有一对如花似玉的双胞胎女儿，姐姐叫小金花，妹妹叫小银花，这一家人乐善好施，深受当地人的爱戴。

有一天，村里突然发生了一场可怕的瘟疫，并很快在全村蔓延。这对小姐妹见村民饮了她们父亲花数日心血配成的解毒汤后仍不能痊愈，被这毒瘟折磨数天后痛苦地死去，便背着父亲，到青龙镇的药神庙前发誓，愿姐妹同心化作良药来解这毒瘟。药神仙便把姐妹二人化作了一株同蒂并开花的植物，托梦给黄神医。第二天一早，黄神医便来到庙前采摘自己孩子化成的花，带回到家里，按神仙的指引煮成茶分给乡亲们喝，果真药到病除。

后来，乡亲们得知救命的药茶是小金花和小银花姐妹用性命换来的，纷纷到药神庙拜谢。为感谢这对善良的小姐妹的救命之恩，乡亲们把那株植物叫作"金银花"，又称"二花"。

传说玉皇大帝得知此义举，甚为感动，就封这对小姐妹为"金银花花仙子"，并让她们永久守护着那片她们热爱的家乡。

猜一猜

古城姐妹。（打一中草药名）

（谜底：金银花）

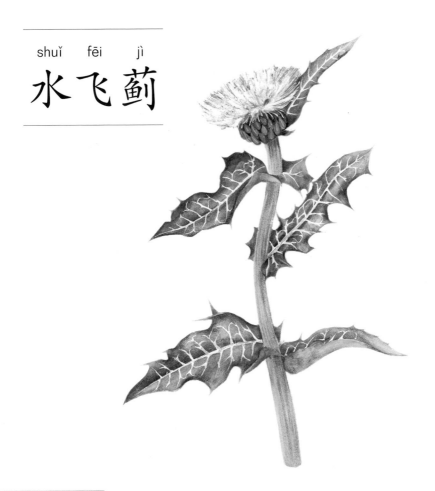

shuǐ fēi jì
水飞蓟

水飞蓟种子发芽温度实验

1. 将采收的新鲜水飞蓟种子放在垫有 4 层纱布的培养皿内做发芽实验，每组 30 粒，分别放在 5~10℃、16~25℃、28~34℃的恒温培养箱内，观察种子的萌发时间及情况。重复 3 次，统计各处理方式下的平均发芽率。

2. 通过实验可知，水飞蓟种子的最适发芽温度为 16~25℃。在 10℃以下或 28℃以上，种子发芽都会受到抑制。在萌发及生长过程中观察到，种子在 16~25℃条件下培养时，第 6 天开始萌发长根，发芽率为 94%。

别名：水飞锥、奶蓟、老鼠筋

拉丁学名：*Silybum marianum*
　　　　　Gaertn.

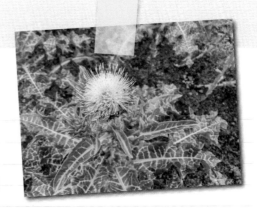

草药小故事 ● **水飞蓟的传说**

　　大约在 20 世纪初期，德国有很多采菇工作者，他们时常到土壤肥沃的山林里采摘菌菇。山里的菌菇种类繁多，多生于山毛榉、栎木和榛木等硬木树上，或者朽木的隐蔽处、被枯叶遮盖的地方。

　　采菇工作者经常会误采一种叫"死亡帽"的剧毒菇。这种菇的菌伞呈绿色或灰色，凸圆形，边缘平滑，表面为内生纤维质，菌褶白色离生，菌柄和菌伞是相同的白色，有显著的菌托，长得和一般无毒菇类很像。误食这种剧毒菇会因肝衰竭而死亡。有不少人因误食这种"死亡帽"而身亡。

　　后来，一位采菇工作者在一次意外中发现食用一种茎直立，分枝，有条棱，开着有花丝的紫色小花朵的草药可以解剧毒菇之毒。这种草药叫作"水飞蓟"，它的枝干切开后会流出类似牛奶般的白色苦味汁液。甚至事先服用了水飞蓟后，再摄食毒菇也不会中毒。这位采菇工作者便把这个好消息告诉了其他采菇工作者，让大家都得到了救治。

　　因为这种草药的枝干被切开后会流出类似牛奶般的白色汁液，所以它也被人们称为"牛奶蓟"。

不可忽略的常识 ● **《本草纲目》里也有错谬？**

　　李时珍编纂《本草纲目》的初衷是纠正过去的本草书籍中的错误，但由于时代局限性，缺乏科学观念和方法，《本草纲目》里仍然有很多荒谬的内容，如喝立春雨水治夫妻不孕不育，吃烧成灰的渔网治鱼刺卡喉，老虎一只眼睛看物一只眼睛放光等，荒唐偏方在其中《人部》《服器部》尤其明显。现今市场的《本草纲目》大多是经过删节处理的，留下的经验疗法（包括偏方）也应通过科学确认其安全性和有效性。

yì mǔ cǎo

益母草

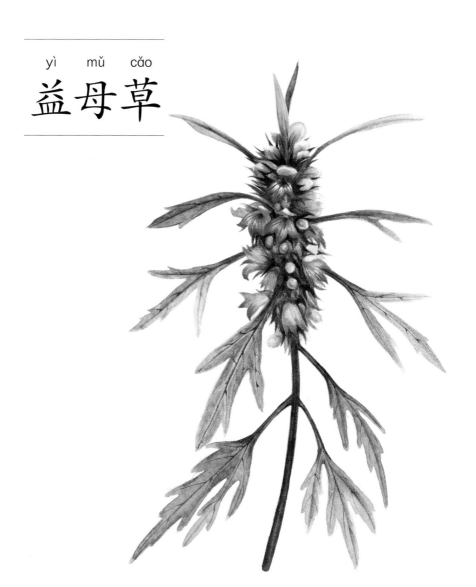

趣味小知识　　**益母草小时候长什么样?**

　　益母草幼小时无茎，基生，心形的圆叶片边上是浅浅的锯齿波浪，叶柄长长的，像打着一把小蒲扇似的，颜色碧绿，很多人又称它"童子草"。

48

别名：益母蒿、益母花、鸡母草
拉丁学名：*Leonurus japonicus* Houttuyn

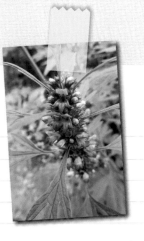

　　益母草的故事

　　古时候，有一个秀才考了几年都没考上，这使他终日郁郁寡欢，饮酒度日。他的母亲因过度担忧他而病倒了，一卧床就是好几个月，请了很多郎中来医治都没好，秀才这下急坏了。

　　有一天，秀才上街看到一个外地来的算命先生，聊天时算命先生告诉他，北城青山脚下有一位医术高明的老人，这位老人或许能够医治他的母亲。这北城青山脚下离他家很远，路途危险，而且也不知道算命先生说的是不是真的，乡亲们都劝他不要去。秀才觉得愧对母亲，无论如何都要把母亲的病治好，安顿好母亲后他就上路了。

　　到了北城青山脚下，果真有一位白发苍苍的老人，老人的院子里晒满了各种草药。秀才说明来意，老人被他的孝心感动，给了他一些草药带回去，并给了他一包种子。秀才谢过老人后就马不停蹄地往家里赶，到家后马上把药煎给母亲服下，不出几天，母亲的病情就好转了。

　　乡亲们纷纷来问秀才这是什么灵丹妙药，秀才就把种子都分给了乡亲们。之后，这个地方的妇女都免受妇科病的困扰。由于这种草是秀才为医治母亲的病而找到的，且有益于妇女，于是人们就叫它"益母草"。

猜一猜

　　一封书慰高堂心。（打一中药名）

（谜底：益母草）

wén shū lán
文殊兰

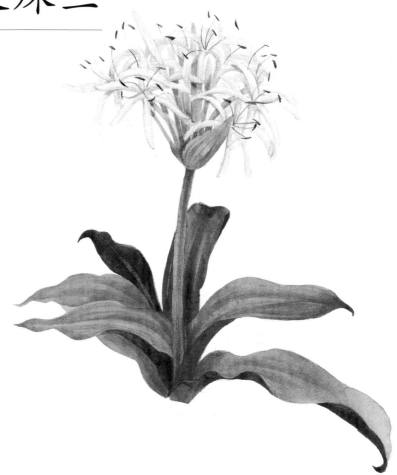

趣味小知识 ◆ **天然的绷带——文殊兰**

　　在深山野林里，迷路又摔伤或者骨折的小朋友可以把文殊兰的叶子摘下，用石头等器具打软后，再用火炙烤，然后就可以拿它当作天然的绷带使用了。

别名：白花石蒜、罗裙带、文兰树
拉丁学名：*Crinum asiaticum* var.
　　　　 sinicum Baker

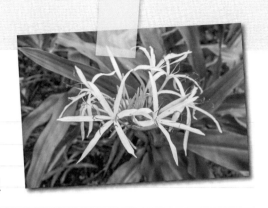

　　文殊兰的传说

　　传说，在公元前6世纪，文殊菩萨是调皮地从他娘亲的右肋钻出来，出生到这个世界上的。文殊菩萨一出生，身体就显现紫金色，不需要学习就会说话，就好像天上的童子一样，身上有七宝盖覆，可以降福于人间。文殊菩萨是智慧的化身，人们把他尊称为"大智文殊师利菩萨"。

　　世界上的所有竞争，其实就是智力的竞争。古希腊有这样一句谚语：从智慧的土壤中生出三片绿叶，一片是好的思想，一片是好的语言，一片是好的行为。用慧眼兰心来形容文殊兰非常恰当。这种美丽的兰花跟佛教非常有因缘，它端坐在佛家寺院里，神情端庄，沾上了文殊菩萨的灵气，显得格外高贵、典雅、美丽，为世人所喜爱。因此，人们将它称为"文殊兰"。

　　盛夏炎热百花稀少之时，文殊兰就盛开了。长长的花梗，撑着伞状的白色花序，显得亭亭玉立，纯洁端庄；丝丝条条的花蕊，散发着愉悦的淡淡香气，带着佛家的灵气，显得大方质朴，似乎告诉我们一定要平心静气，拂去心中的烦躁和焦虑。

猜一猜

　　空谷佳人恋君子，淡淡清香夜夜思（打一植物名）

（谜底：兰花）

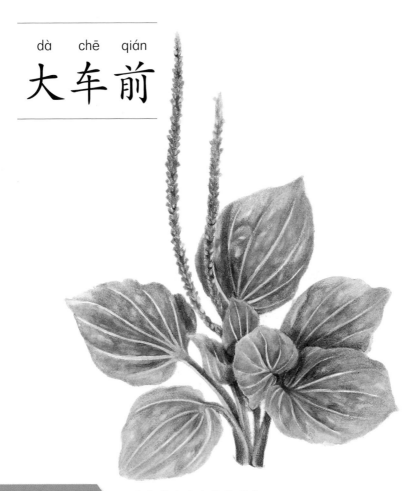

dà chē qián
大车前

大车前和小车前的形态

大车前：（1）多年生草本；（2）根状茎短粗，有须根；（3）叶直立，叶片卵形或宽卵形，顶端圆钝，边缘波状或有不整齐锯齿；（4）花茎直立，高 15~120 厘米；（5）蒴果椭圆形；（6）种子 8~18 粒，呈棕色或棕褐色。

小车前：（1）一年生草本；（2）圆柱状直根；（3）叶直立或平铺，叶片椭圆形、椭圆状披针形或卵状披针形；（4）花弧曲，长 4~17 厘米；（5）蒴果圆锥状；（6）种子呈黑棕色。

别名：钱贯草、大叶车前、大猪耳朵草
拉丁学名：*Plantago major* L.

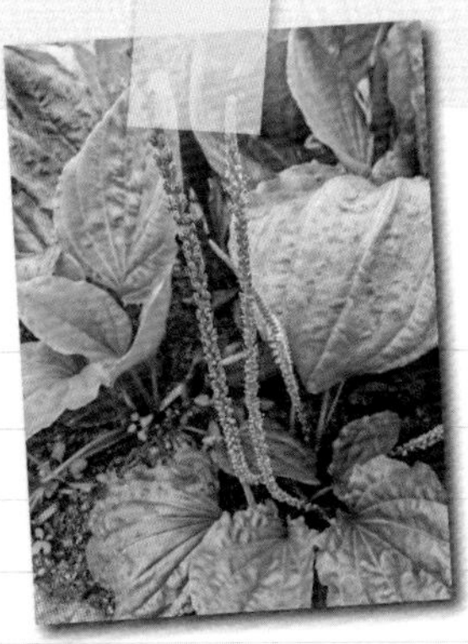

车前草的故事

西汉时有一位名将叫马武。有一次，马武带领军队去边境征战，被敌军围困在一个荒无人烟的地方。当时酷热异常，又干旱无雨。由于缺食少水，士兵和战马饿死、渴死的不少。剩下的士兵也因饥渴交加，肚子胀得很大，痛苦不堪，小便时刺痛难忍，尿像血一样红。战马拉尿时也嘶鸣挣扎。军医诊断为尿血症，需要清热利水的药物来治疗。因为没有药物，军医都束手无策。

马武有一个马夫，名叫张勇。张勇和他分管的三匹马也同样患了尿血症，人和马都十分痛苦。

有一天，张勇发现他的三匹马都不尿血了，马的精神也大为好转。他便紧盯着马的活动，发现马一天都在啃食附近地面上一种酷似猪耳朵的野草。于是他拔了一些草，捣汁煎水一连服了几天，感觉身体舒服了，小便也正常了。

张勇把这个偶然的发现报告给马武。马武非常高兴，立即号令全军吃"猪耳朵草"。几天之后，士兵和马都好转了。

因为此草是在车前面发现的，所以人们叫它"车前草"。

猜一猜 ●

马上相逢无纸笔。（打一中草药）

（谜底：车前草）

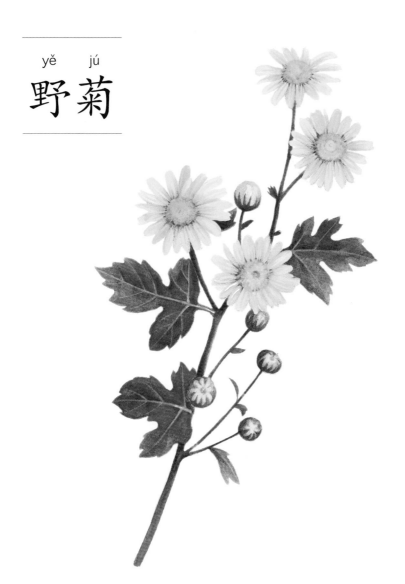

野菊

yě jú

小朋友，你知道野菊的美吗？

野菊有一种朴实的美。野菊生长于山野，花色清淡，香气沁人心脾。野菊在秋天开花，人们常借野菊来表现不与世俗同流合污、坚贞不屈的高尚品格。

别名：黄菊仔、路边黄、山菊花
拉丁学名：*Chrysanthemum indicum* L.

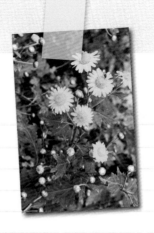

　　　　野菊的故事

　　过去，在一条叫鲁河的边上，住着一个叫阿牛的人。阿牛的父亲在他七岁的时候就过世了，他的母亲靠织布养活他，非常辛苦，再加上心疼孩子自小就没有父亲，母亲经常哭，最后把眼睛都哭瞎了。

　　阿牛长大了，每日去卖菜挣钱给他母亲治眼睛。花了很多钱，买了很多药给母亲吃，可是母亲的眼睛却一直没有治好。

　　有一天晚上，阿牛梦见一个漂亮的姑娘，姑娘被阿牛的孝心感动了，她让他到山里的某一个地方去找一棵野菊，那棵野菊的花可以治好他母亲的病。阿牛醒后，立刻出发去寻找梦里的野菊。

　　他来到梦中姑娘说的那个地方，一直找到下午，才终于找到了那棵野菊。野菊一个梗上有九个花头，但是只开了一朵，阿牛就把它连土带根搬回了家。阿牛每天都细心地照料着野菊，给野菊浇水，慢慢地，花儿都开了。他就每天摘一朵花给母亲煮一杯茶喝，喝到第八天的时候，母亲的眼睛居然能看到东西了。

　　从这个故事中，我们可以看到野菊的花具有明目的功效。

猜一猜

　　重阳花满枝。（打一中草药）

（答案：野菊）

钉头果

dīng tóu guǒ

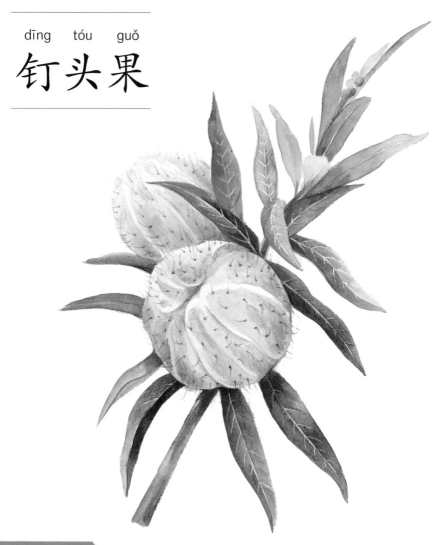

趣味小知识 ● **奇特的果实——钉头果**

　　钉头果呈黄绿色，果面有刺突，果实很薄，中心是空的，肿胀呈球形，用手轻轻挤压，似有空气溢出，极像小气球。果实挂在枝头很长时间都不会掉落，可作盆栽观赏植物。

别名：气球花、气球果、棒头果
拉丁学名：*Gomphocarpus fruticosus*
W. T. Ation

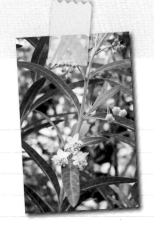

　　　钉头果的故事

　　千百年前，传说神秘的地中海上有一个很漂亮的岛屿。岛屿上夏天炎热干燥，冬天温暖湿润，长满绿灌木，盛产丰富的亚热带水果。

　　岛上有一户犹太人常常出海经商，由于父母太忙，4 岁的弟弟就交由 10 岁的哥哥看护。哥哥常常带着弟弟到林子里采摘水果。嘴馋的弟弟经常在小路上随手摘一些奇怪的果实放到嘴里吃。

　　由于什么果实都往嘴里塞，回到家里，弟弟不停地拉肚子。看着因拉肚子而脸色发青的弟弟，哥哥被吓坏了。

　　不停拉肚子的弟弟虽然很难受，但是肚子也因拉的次数过多而饿得"咕噜噜"地叫起来，他看到自己在路上摘的、放桌上的那长有软刺的果实，便拿来往嘴里塞。

　　吓呆的哥哥没能及时阻止弟弟又乱吃东西。可是弟弟吃了之后，停止了腹泻，脸蛋也开始恢复了红润。这种植物的果子实长相奇怪、带有软刺，好像长了钉子一样，于是，他们就把这种植物的果实叫作"钉头果"。

猜一猜

　　黄绿果子长软刺，两指一捏就泄气。（打一植物名）

（谜底：钉头果）

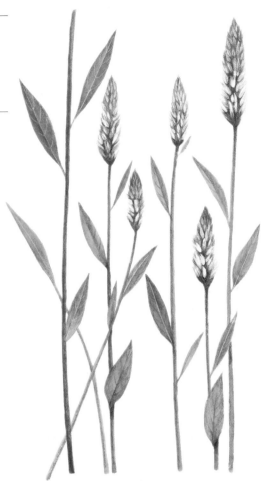

qīng xiāng
青葙

小朋友，你知道青葙的种子长什么样吗？
我们一起来观察吧！

青葙子是植物青葙的种子，在 8~10 月采收，割取地上部分或者花穗，晒干；然后从花穗里搓出种子，除去杂质，晒干。

干燥的青葙子呈扁圆形，中心较边缘稍厚，直径 1~1.5 毫米，厚约 0.5 毫米，表面平滑，黑色，有光泽。种子的皮薄而脆，容易破碎，里面是白色，有微微的臭味。

别名：野鸡冠花、鸡冠花、百日红
拉丁学名：*Celosia argentea* L.

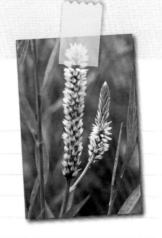

青葙子的故事

相传，有一位猎人，每天都会到山林里打猎。

有一天，猎人像往常一样去山林里打猎，突然隐隐约约听到山林里传来哭声。他循着声音搜寻过去，看到草丛中放着一个青色的大箱子。猎人警觉起来，慢慢地靠近大箱子，然后，猎人打开箱子的盖子，发现里面蜷缩着一个衣衫破烂的姑娘。

猎人好心救起姑娘，把姑娘带回家梳洗，询问姑娘为什么会在山林里的大箱子里面。原来，姑娘的母亲得了一种眼病，有一天，山村里来了两个自称是游医的男子，姑娘就请他们到家里给母亲治病。两个游医胡乱为姑娘的母亲看了眼睛后说，要上山去采一些药给姑娘的母亲治病，便让姑娘带路。上山后，两个歹人把姑娘关进箱子里，还未来得及运走，就被猎人发现了。

猎人把姑娘送回家，随即采来野鸡冠花种子煎出汤水，一部分让姑娘的母亲服用，一部分用来洗眼睛。不久，姑娘母亲的眼睛就治好了。

山村里的人因为这件事，从此便把野鸡冠花叫"青葙"，它的种子便叫"青葙子"了。

奇怪野公鸡，天天站这里，
晚上不进笼，白天也不啼。（打一花卉名）

（谜底：鸡冠花）

59

shǔ kuí

蜀葵

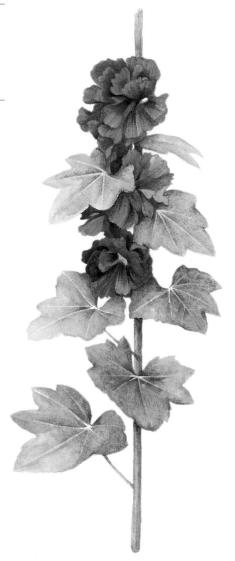

趣味小知识

蜀葵为什么又叫"一丈红"?

蜀葵是山西省朔州市市花,它的花朵大,花期长,当地人称它"大花"。因为蜀葵高可达 3 米,花多为红色,所以又称"一丈红"。

别名：一丈红、麻秆花、斗篷花
拉丁学名：*Alcea rosea* L.

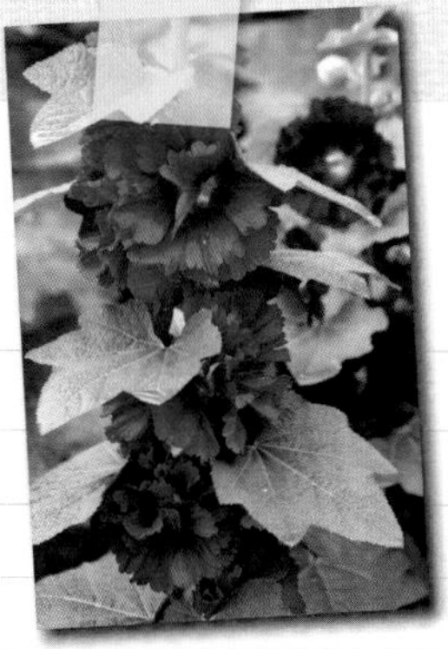

蜀葵的传说

相传古时候有一个员外，家里还算富裕，对待佣人十分和善。员外娶了一个非常美丽、娇弱的妻子蜀葵，妻子温和贤惠，员外对她非常疼惜。

可惜，员外妻子的身体一直不好。尽管员外细心呵护，妻子的身体还是越来越虚弱，两年后便去世了。

员外因此伤痛欲绝，整日把自己关在房间，茶饭不思。因思念爱妻，员外整个人都消瘦了，佣人看到都心疼不已。有一天晚上，妻子托梦给员外，说她会幻化成花儿一直陪在员外的身边，不离不弃。

梦醒后，员外急忙跑到院子里，只见院子里长了一株茎直立而高，有心脏形叶子的植物，细瘦的茎上密匝匝地开满非常美丽的花儿。花盘硕大，颜色十分艳丽，就像妻子生前一样娇艳动人。这些花朝开暮落，但这丝毫不影响它毫无保留地绽放自己。阵阵凉风吹拂着轻轻摇摆的花儿，似乎是妻子在对他点头微笑。

之后的日子里，员外把花当作妻子一样细心照料。第二年，院子里都长满了这种花儿，满院的芬芳。为了纪念妻子，员外给花儿取了和妻子一样的名字——蜀葵。

猜一猜

为革命而死重于泰山。（打一花卉名）

（谜底：一丈红）

61

wǔ yuè ài
五月艾

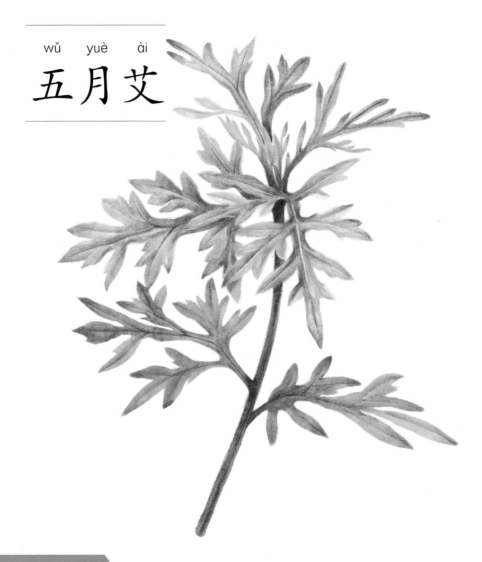

为什么端午要插艾?

　　艾草代表招百福,是一种可以治病的药草,插在门口,可让人身体健康。

　　我国民间历来就广泛利用艾草,有的用它来治病,有的用它来充饥,更有的用它来辟邪驱毒。

别名：艾、野艾蒿、艾叶
拉丁学名：*Artemisia indica* Willd.

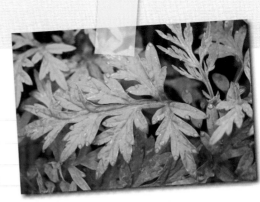

草药小故事　　　　**五月艾的故事**

　　有一年，风调雨顺，一位天神变成一个衣衫褴褛的白胡子老爷爷来察看民情。他走进一户人家，看到桌上都是剩饭，便向前讨吃，却被妇人赶了出去。

　　老爷爷心里恼怒，用手指冲着大门比画了一阵，门上出现了两行大字：明日起瘟病，全村人死净。妇人这才知道自己的无知闯了大祸，悔恨不已，乡亲们知道后也都责怪她。

　　第二天清早，天神正准备向村子撒瘟药，忽见村头小河里有一个妇人怀里抱着一个大孩子，手里牵着一个小孩子蹚着河水往对岸走。

　　他觉得十分奇怪，便落下云头去询问。

　　妇人叹气解释道，村子准备来瘟疫了，她带着两个孩子逃命。因为大孩子是她丈夫的前妻留下的，不忍让他蹚水便抱着了。

　　老头敬佩地点了点头，从地上拔了棵五月艾，让妇人插在窗上或门上。

　　说完，他用手一指，河面上立即出现了一座大桥。那妇人才知道遇见了神仙，便接过五月艾谢恩，随后带着两个孩子拔了一大捆五月艾，顺着神仙点化的大桥过了河。他们赶回村子，在每家每户的门窗上都插上一棵五月艾。

　　村子里的乡亲们得救了，都来感谢那位插五月艾的妇人。

猜一猜

　　风流几度苦别离。（打一中药名）

（谜底：艾叶）

63

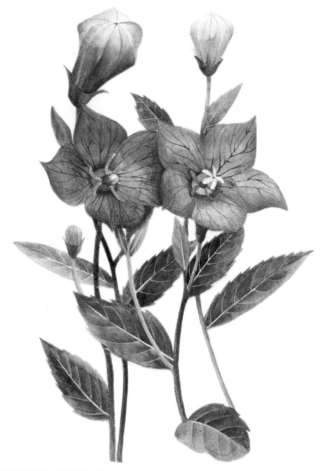

jié   gěng
桔梗

桔梗是如何过冬的?

桔梗因花形似僧帽而得别名"僧冠帽",又因似荷花而别称"六角荷"。桔梗是一种深根性植物,根的直径会随年龄的增大而增大,根可在地下越冬,过完冬,第二年会从老根处萌发出新芽。而它的苗可在−17℃的低温下安全越冬。

桔梗一年能开两次花吗?

如果想让桔梗每年开两次花,可以在它第一次开花后,于7月底之前进行修剪,并加强肥水管理,及时预防和治理病虫害,10月初桔梗就会再次开花。

别名：铃铛花、包袱花、僧帽花
拉丁学名：*Platycodon grandiflorus* A. DC.

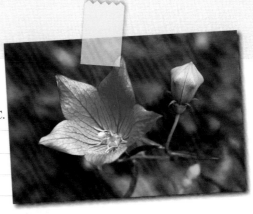

桔梗的传说

传说，在某个村子里住着一位叫桔梗的少女。桔梗没有父母，独自一人生活。

村里有一个天天来找桔梗玩的少年，少年对桔梗说："桔梗啊，长大了我要跟你结婚。"桔梗很高兴，说："我长大了也要跟你结婚。"两人就这样约好了。

几年后，桔梗长成了漂亮的小姑娘，少年也长成了英俊的小伙子，两人成了一对恋人。但是，小伙子为了捕鱼，不得不乘大船去很远的地方。

桔梗深爱着的小伙子，十年了也没回来。桔梗每天都到海边等小伙子，她越看大海越伤心。

就这样过了几十年，桔梗已经成了老人，她每次看到大海总会想起回不来的恋人，不禁流下眼泪。

"祈求上苍，一定要让我心爱的他回来。"

这时，神灵现身了："你苦等难受，所以，现在我要你放弃这份思念。"

"神灵，不管怎样，我的心不变啊！"

神灵叹了口气道："不是让你放弃这份思念了吗？我要给你定下不能忘掉恋人的罪。"

于是，桔梗的眼睛慢慢地闭上，身体变成了花。

后来，人们就把那朵花叫作"桔梗花"，桔梗花一直看着大海，等待着小伙子。

洞房花烛夜。（打一中药名）

（谜底：桔梗，即新婚的意思。）

cháng chūn huā

长春花

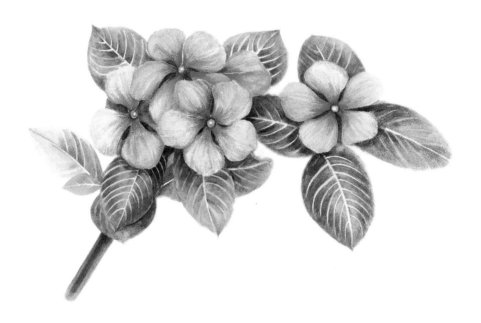

趣味小知识 ●　　**有毒的长春花**

　　长春花的嫩枝顶端，每长出一片叶子，叶腋间就冒出两朵花，因此它的花朵特别多。又因为它从春天到秋天不间断地开花，所以有着"日日春"之美名。长春花的乳汁中所含的生物碱，如长春花碱和长春新碱，可提炼出来作为治疗多种癌症如白血病、霍奇金病等的化学药物，被医者配入治疗癌症的复方。但长春花全株具毒性，误食后，会出现白细胞减少、血小板减少、肌肉无力、四肢麻痹等症状。

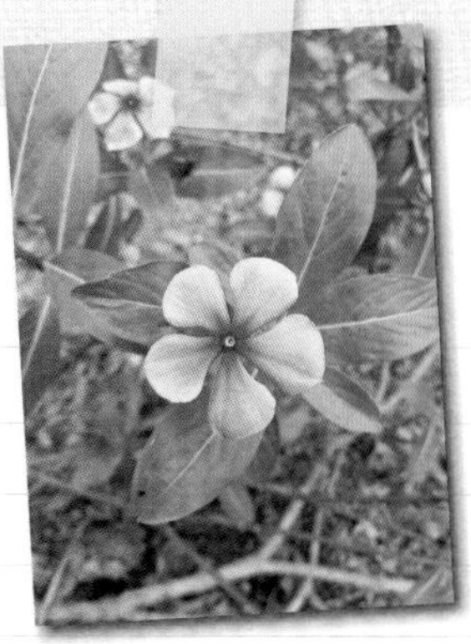

别名：雁来红、日日新、日日春
拉丁学名：*Catharanthus roseus* G. Don

梅绽坡的故事

江西九江有个地方叫作梅绽坡，传说这个地名的由来跟长春花有关。

清代崇德年间，有一个多年在外经商的梅姓商人，回浔定居，并在坡前的街口开了一家布店。他平时待人真诚，做生意也不斤斤计较，大家都喜欢到他那里买布匹。

这位梅姓商人平时除了打理生意，还喜欢花草。为了纪念初恋情人，他便在房前屋后种了数十株初恋情人喜欢的长春花（老百姓称之为"四季梅"），他还特地在店铺门口也种了两排。长春花属于蔓生类花草，一旦开始生长，就繁殖得很快，能长满整个庭院。而且这种花的花朵特别多，花期特别长，花势繁茂，生机勃勃。到了秋天，百花凋谢，而他的四季梅却依然开得那么耀眼，即使冬天也是如此。附近的居民见了，也都喜爱不已，纷纷前来索种。梅姓商人心地善良，慷慨地把花种分给每一个前来索取的村民。

那些生意经营不下去的商人认为，梅家店铺之所以这么红火，是这长春花带来的好运，于是，也纷纷学习梅姓商人，在自家店门口种上了这种花。一时间，大街小巷，梅花绽放。"梅绽坡"由此得名。

人送外号雁来红，提炼出来抗病痛。（打一花卉名）

（谜底：长春花）

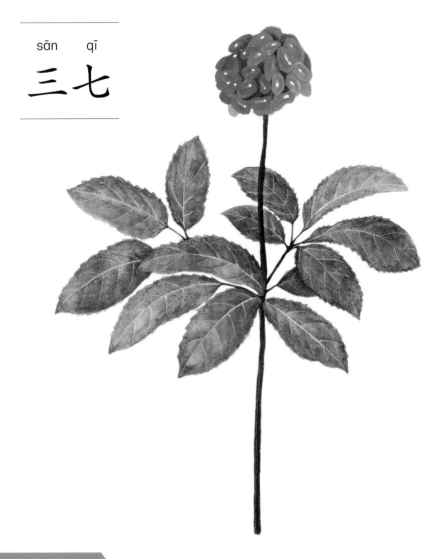

sān qī

三七

趣味小知识 **你认识三七吗？**

　　三七又名"田七"，自古以来就因其显著的散瘀止血、消肿止痛功效而有"南国神草""金不换"之美誉，又因常在春冬两季采挖，分为"春七"和"冬七"。

别名：田七、金不换、血见愁
拉丁学名：*Panax notoginseng* F. H. Chen ex C. H. Chow

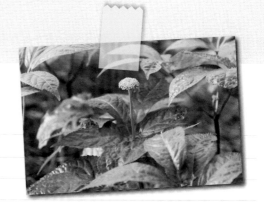

三七的传说

相传，有一位美丽善良的三七仙子来到人间教人们种植作物。

有一天，三七仙子在地里劳作时，突然有一只凶猛的大黑熊朝她扑来。在这千钧一发之际，一位名叫卡相的苗族青年，一箭射死了这只猛兽，救了三七仙子。

卡相家里很穷，他的母亲患病多年，无钱医治。三七仙子为报卡相的救命之恩，对卡相说："后山坡有一种草药，叶像我的长裙，枝似我的腰带，可以用来治疗你母亲的病。"卡相按其所说，果真找到了这种草药。他的母亲吃了几次这种草药后，病真的好了。

后来，卡相又用这种草药治好了不少乡亲们的疾病。

乡亲们纷纷来到卡相家道谢，并问："这是什么药？怎么这么神奇？"

三七仙子笑盈盈地指着一株三七说："你们数数看，它枝有多少？叶有多少？"

大家一数，枝有三根，叶有七片。

一个聪明的姑娘立即叫了起来："三七！"这个名字从此就流传了下来。

猜一猜

两字相乘二十一。（打一中药名）

妇女节的前一天。（打一中药名）

（答案：三七）

大叶仙茅

dà yè xiān máo

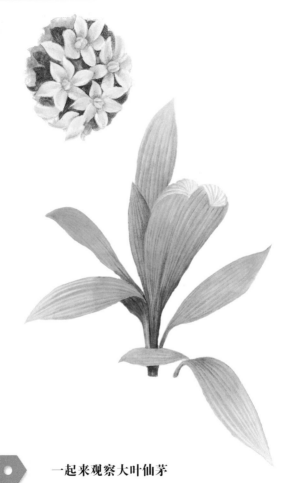

一起来观察大叶仙茅

把大叶仙茅的根茎种在花盆里，看看它什么时候开花？开出什么颜色的花？

别名：独茅根、野棕、假槟榔树
拉丁学名：*Curculigo capitulata* O. Kuntze

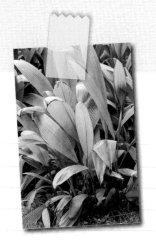

大叶仙茅的由来

　　唐代皇帝李世民为了长生不老，吃了很多药，但是，无论他每天吃多少，还是一天天地衰老。

　　于是，李世民很不满意，就昭告天下：谁能找到一种长生不老的药，就重赏谁。这个消息很快传遍了全国，并且传到了西域各国。有一天，来了一个西域使者，他将一种形如大蒜的东西作为仙药，进贡给了李世民。李世民服用仙药后感到精神抖擞、体力大增，感觉像回到年轻时候一样。大臣们也个个惊叹皇帝重返年轻，纷纷想知道这是什么神药。

　　于是，李世民把西域使者招来，西域使者说："其叶似茅，像神仙生长在隐蔽的地方，叫仙茅。"

　　李世民设宴重赏了这位西域使者之后，把仙茅作为禁药藏于宫中，不准外传，以独自享用。

　　直到唐代开元年间，唐僧得到此方，仙茅才流传到民间。

　　灵芝草。（打一中药名）

　　　　　　　　　　　　　　　（谜底：大叶仙茅）

kǔ　shēn

苦参

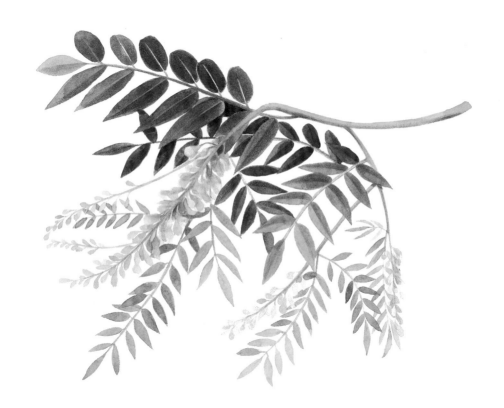

趣味小知识 ▶　　**苦参名字的由来**

　　小朋友们，知道苦参为什么叫"苦参"吗？尝一尝，是不是很苦呀？告诉你们一个秘密，因为苦参味道很苦，形状像人参，所以就叫它"苦参"。

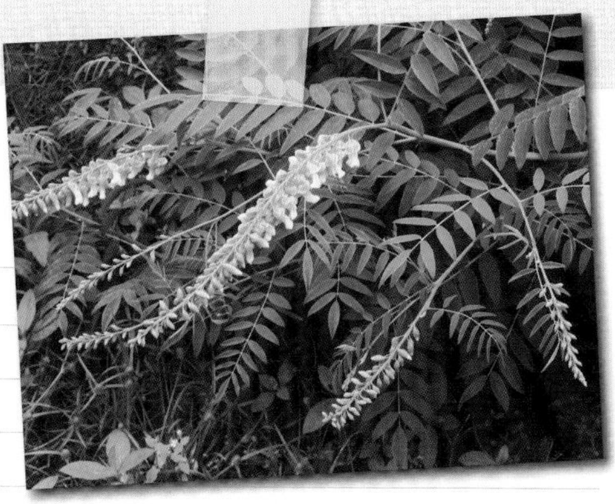

别名：地槐、白茎地骨、山槐
拉丁学名：*Sophora flavescens* Ait.

　　苦参的故事

很久以前，有一个放牛娃，他爹妈去世得早，他以给地主放牛为生。由于经常在湿地上行走，放牛娃身上长满了疮。

不久，地主家里人的身上也长满了疮。大家都说疮是放牛娃传染的，于是，地主就下令追杀放牛娃。

放牛娃只能逃命，他躲到大山的一个石缝里，再也没出来。后来，村民发现放牛娃的时候，他已经死了。好心的村民就用泥沙和石头把石缝封住，算是给放牛娃一个死后的安身之地。

不久，村民身上也长了疮，奇痒无比，试了很多药都治不好。一天晚上，大家都梦见了放牛娃，放牛娃告诉村民，在当初埋他的山体塌方处有许多根状物，把这些根状物拿回家熬水喝或用来洗澡，身上的疮就会消退。村民按照梦中放牛娃的提示去做，不出几日，身上的疮果然都消退了。

地主听说村民吃了山体塌方处的草药后，疮很快就消退了，于是他也去那个地方采药。看到岩石上灌木丛中结满如老鼠屎粒大小的果子，地主就赶紧摘回家熬水喝，谁知当晚就断肠而死。

原来，村民们吃的是苦参的根，而地主吃的却是苦参子，这是另一种植物鸦胆子的果子，这个果子是有毒的。

谋士难当。（打一中药名）

（谜底：苦参）

73

lóng yá cǎo

龙牙草

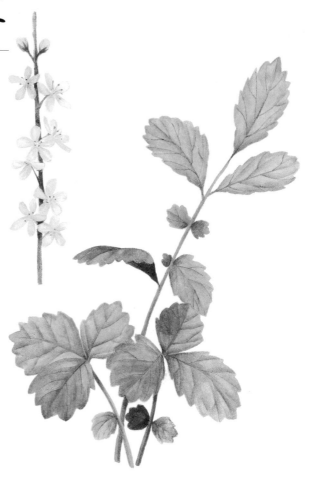

仙鹤草止血有奇效

　　龙牙草也叫"仙鹤草"。仙鹤草有很好的止血作用，因此，当我们在野外摔伤出血或者不小心划伤的时候，可以将仙鹤草揉搓后敷在伤口上，伤口很快就会停止流血了。

别名：仙鹤草、脱力草、老鹳嘴
拉丁学名：*Agrimonia pilosa* Ledeb.

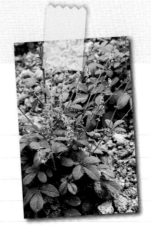

止血良药仙鹤草

传说古时候，两个举人进京赶考，途中路过一片沙滩。正好是盛夏，烈日当空，他们被晒得汗流浃背，又渴又累。

这时，一个举人流鼻血，另一个慌了手脚。在荒郊野外，一无医，二无药，他们只好看着鲜红的血从那位举人的鼻子中流出。正在他俩焦急的时候，只见一只仙鹤嘴里衔着几棵草，慢慢从他们头顶飞过来，在上空把几棵草扔下，草刚好落在他们面前。流鼻血的举人急忙把野草放在嘴里嚼了起来，有了水分的滋润，举人的嗓子不干了，口也不渴了，没一会儿，鼻血也不流了。他们非常高兴，急忙继续赶路。

后来，他们都中了进士，当了七品县官，但难忘这段奇特的经历，于是派人到山上寻找那种能止鼻血的野草。这种野草经医者辨认试验，证实它确实有止血的功效。

为纪念送草药的仙鹤，他们就把这种野草取名叫"仙鹤草"，仙鹤草从而流传民间，并载入书中，广为药用。

猜一猜

神鸟落地变百草。（打一中药名）

（谜底：仙鹤草）

葫芦茶
hú lu chá

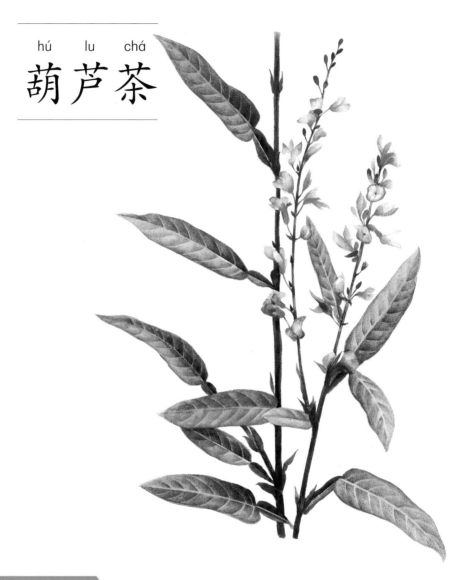

巧记葫芦茶

　　小朋友，你看葫芦茶的叶子像什么呀？一大一小的两片叶子长在一起像不像一个葫芦？以后见到这种植物，一看叶子就知道它叫什么了吧？

别名：百劳舌、牛虫草、懒狗舌
拉丁学名：*Tadehagi triquetrum* Ohashi

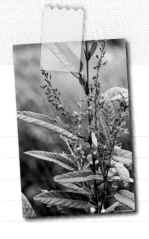

　　葫芦茶的故事

　　很久很久以前，有一个挑鱼的挑夫，趁夜里凉快，走了几十里旱路，把一担鱼卖给了约定的买主。

　　第二天回家，碰上大热天，太阳毒得像热锅扣在头顶。挑夫好不容易坚持走到了山岗下面，看到有一户农舍。农舍里有一棵大树，树底下有一位老婆婆正坐着绩麻。

　　他走过去向老婆婆讨水喝，老婆婆二话没说，转身进屋端出一碗凉茶："年轻人，这一碗够你喝吧？"

　　挑夫连忙说谢谢，接过凉茶咕噜噜一口气把那一大碗凉茶喝得精光。挑夫顿时觉得浑身有劲儿，先前的难受完全消失了。为了感谢老婆婆，挑夫从裢裢里掏出一个铜板，递给老婆婆。

　　老婆婆瞥了挑夫一眼，没有伸手接他那块铜板，对他说："年轻人，我们家的凉茶是不要钱的，我们一天煮一罐，自家人喝，也给过路人喝。"

　　挑夫只好收起那块铜板，连声向老婆婆道谢，临走前询问老婆婆凉茶是用什么煮的。老婆婆眼皮一抬，指着屋旁的一棵叶子像葫芦一样的植物跟他说："就是这个，叫葫芦茶！"

　　挑夫回去后把这件事告诉了乡亲们，就这样，用葫芦茶做凉茶的方法就流传开了。

猜一猜

　　小小植物立着走，叶像葫芦果像豆，能当茶来能做药。（打一植物名）

（谜底：葫芦茶）

guǎng xī dì bù róng

广西地不容

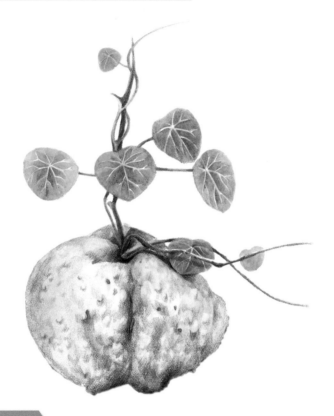

趣味小知识 ▶ **广西地不容名字的由来**

　　长在地面上的"大球球"是广西地不容的根，因为它是多年生落叶藤本植物，根部长有肉质块根，因块根越长越大，地里容不下就长到地上来，所以叫"地不容"。地不容可以作盆景，深受人们的喜爱。它可以土栽也可以水培，水培很简单，只需把块根底部的根须浸入水中就行了。

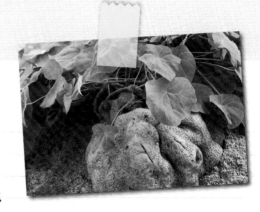

别名：山乌龟、金不换、地胆
拉丁学名：*Stephania kwangsiensis* H. S. Lo.

　　山乌龟的传说

相传，古时候，在我国南方有一个小国叫野王国。

有一年夏天，野王国和大国交战。野王国人少，自然打不过人多的大国。败仗之后逃到深山里，途中，士兵们带着伤一路跌倒，身上又肿又痛，十分难受。又因天气暑热，很多士兵在林子里得了湿疹，且又肚子痛又腹泻，纷纷倒下了。

在绝望之际，一位士兵抱着从地面挖来的一个又大又圆、形状像乌龟一样的东西，说自己小时候听说这个东西有毒，想着现在没办法了，就吃了一点试一下，想以毒攻毒，结果还真有效。这名士兵不但腹泻停止了，身上也不痒了，疼痛也消退了。

将军就命令士兵们把那个大块头的肉质圆球状的东西磨碎，撒一点到食物里面给大家吃。几天之后，士兵们都不腹泻了，身上也不痒了，而且很多士兵身上的肿痛也奇迹般地消失了。

大家都认为是老天爷在帮他们，顿时精神焕发，体力大增。将军一声令下，士兵们如猛虎一般冲出山林，夺回失地，保住了国家。

因为它膨大的根长在地面上，形状像乌龟，后来将士们为了纪念这种植物，就给它取名叫"山乌龟"。

猜一猜

什么植物，土也掩埋不了它？（打一植物名）

（谜底：地不容）

luò   dì   shēng   gēn

落地生根

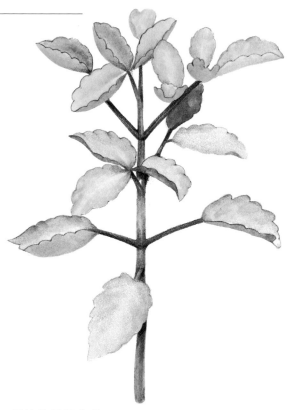

▶ **落地生根的由来**

　　小朋友，你知道它为什么叫"落地生根"吗？这种植物的生命力很强，它的叶片只要落到地上，就会很快生根发芽。不如我们来做个实验：取一片它的叶子放在花盆里，过几天，观察一下有什么变化。是不是发现从叶子的边缘长出了许多的小根呀？这还不算奇怪，更让人惊喜的是，长根的地方会冒出许多许多的新芽，每一棵新芽都是一个新的落地生根小宝宝哦。

别名：打不死草、叶生根、晒不死
拉丁学名：*Bryophyllum pinnatum* Oken

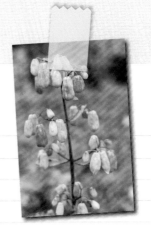

　　　　顽强的生命力——打不死草

　　传说，从前有一对很相爱的青年男女。可是头领看中了美丽的姑娘，派人送去厚礼，要姑娘嫁给他。姑娘不肯，头领一怒之下就带人抢走了姑娘。抢到姑娘后，头领用各种厚礼诱惑姑娘，姑娘就是不为所动。姑娘坚贞不渝，最后竟以死明志。

　　小伙子知道后非常悲痛，擦干眼泪对着姑娘坟前的小草发誓，一定要为姑娘讨回公道。没过多久，小伙子果然做到了，为姑娘讨回了公道。待他又回到姑娘坟前时，没想到竟出现了奇迹，只见坟地周围全都长满了一种小草，并且坟头裂开，姑娘从中走了出来。于是，他们俩又重逢了。

　　不久，他们就在当地消失了。后来，有人说曾经在遥远的他乡看见过他们。他们到处给人治病，特别擅长治筋骨疼痛、跌打损伤，连骨头断裂都能接好如初。他们给人治病用的药就是姑娘坟头长出的"打不死草"。

　　四季常绿叶，落地就生根。街上有人卖，盆里可种它。（打一植物名）

（谜底：落地生根）

81

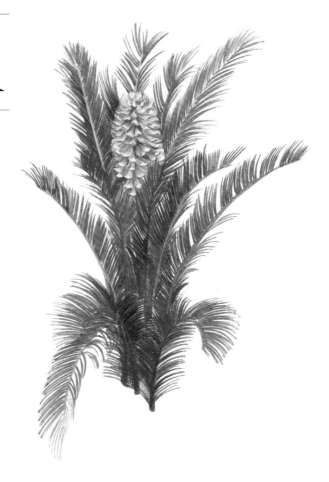

sū tiě
苏铁

怎样区分雄苏铁和雌苏铁？

　　苏铁的树干就像铁一样坚硬，并且喜欢含有微量元素铁的肥料，所以被人们称为"铁树"。苏铁是雌雄异株的植物，那么怎样区分哪棵是雄的，哪棵是雌的呢？很简单，看它开在茎干顶端的花，雄花像个大玉米棒子，雌花像个大包菜。

　　苏铁不仅是优美的观赏树种，还是药食两用的宝贝。它的茎内含淀粉，可以食用；种子含油和丰富的淀粉，微毒，可供食用和药用。

别名：铁树、辟火蕉、凤尾草、凤尾蕉
拉丁学名：*Cycas revoluta* Thunb.

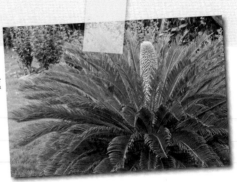

草药小故事　　　**铁树的由来**

相传，很久以前，我国南方住着一只金凤凰，它不但羽毛美丽耀眼，而且还有一副好歌喉。

金凤凰有时立于树梢，有时盘旋于空中，给辛勤劳作的百姓唱着动听的歌儿，展示优雅的舞姿，深受百姓的喜爱。

有一位官员听说了这只金凤凰的事，他非常想独自占有这只金凤凰。于是，官员就派人把它捉住，关在笼子里，给它喂最好、最美味的食物，用尽一切方法讨好金凤凰，想让金凤凰展开它那美丽的羽毛，或者唱歌、跳舞供他欣赏。可金凤凰就是不展羽毛，更是不唱也不跳。

时间一久，官员被惹怒了，他再也没有耐心等下去，于是就点了一把火把金凤凰活活烧死了。

大火熄灭后，在遗留的灰烬中，竟然长出了一棵小树，这小树的叶片如同金凤凰的尾巴，但是非常坚硬，而且是深绿色的。

人们认为这是那只金凤凰变成的，都十分钦佩它那宁死不屈的精神，于是给小树取名为"铁树"。又因为小树的形状非常像金凤凰的尾巴，所以又称它为"凤尾蕉"。

猜一猜

树干硬如铁，树叶美如凤，喜光开花难。（打一植物名）

（答案：铁树）

83

tiě pí shí hú
铁皮石斛

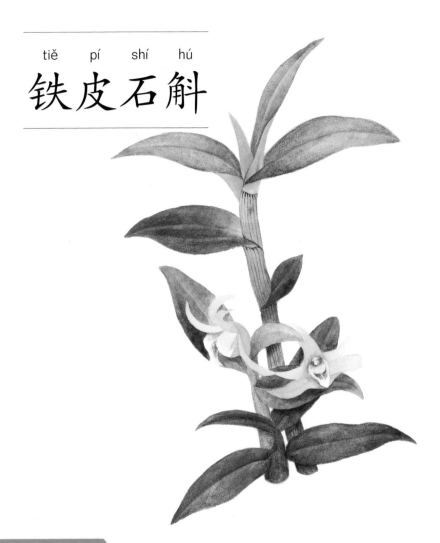

趣味小知识 ● **食用铁皮石斛都有哪些好处呢？**

1. 可以滋阴保健、延年益寿。

2. 女性食用可以美容、滋养皮肤。

3. 适合缓解因压力过大、工作过劳、熬夜加班导致的身体疲劳。

4. 适合缓解因体液循环不佳引起的便秘、痤疮、口干舌燥。

别名：老枫斗、铁皮兰、岩竹
拉丁学名：*Dendrobium catenatum* Lindl.

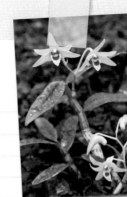

草药小故事

铁皮石斛的故事

很久以前，有一个皇帝，他每天都在寻找能长生不老的药。有一天，皇帝身边的一个小道士向皇帝报告，说他做了一个梦，梦见神仙下凡跟他说话。皇帝感到好奇，便询问小道士做了什么梦。小道士说他在梦里来到一个地方，那里有广阔无边的大海，海边有一座高山，上面飘着很多羽毛。小道士在那里站了一段时间，随着羽毛越积越多，一位白衣仙子出现了。

一开始，小道士十分兴奋，白衣仙子也很和善。白衣仙子感慨自己和小道士的缘分，赠予小道士一棵淡紫色的植物后就离开了。正当小道士拿着手中的植物百思不得其解时，一只巨大的蛟龙出现了，小道士吓得差点晕过去。

这时，蛟龙张开血盆巨口，冲着小道士大喊："你这等小人物，也配拿着你手中的宝物？那可是用来解百毒、令人起死回生的仙草，凡夫俗子怎么配拥有，快放下！"说着蛟龙拿走了小道士手中的植物。小道士也被蛟龙吓得从梦中惊醒过来。

其实小道士梦中所出现的植物就是铁皮石斛。了解到铁皮石斛原来还有这样一个有趣的神话故事，当你在食用它的时候，是不是也增添了一些乐趣呢？

猜一猜

生津之最。（打一药材名）

（谜底：石斛）

shí wéi
石韦

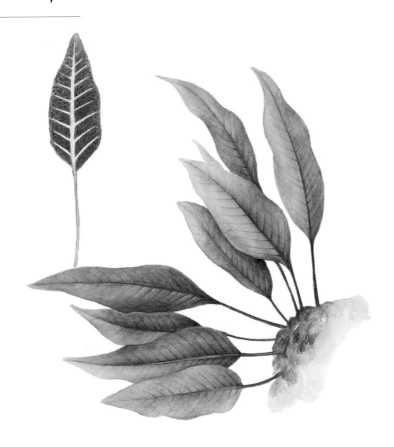

石韦叶背面的秘密

　　石韦是中型附生蕨类植物，植株可高达 30 厘米。它的茎是横走的根状，叶片表面是灰绿色。如果你把叶背翻过来看一看，会发现有很多淡棕色或近砖红色的粉末状东西，这些就是石韦的孢子囊群，里面住着它的"小宝宝"们。

别名：石皮、石苇、石剑
拉丁学名：*Pyrrosia lingua* Farwell

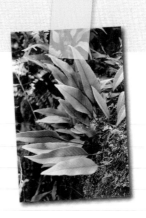

草药小故事　　　**石韦的由来**

　　传说，《史记》的作者司马迁早年在宫廷当吏官，主要记录帝王的生活起居以及朝政大事。帝王只许司马迁颂其功勋而非过错，可司马迁经常不思变通，屡次得罪帝王。加之李陵叛变之事，司马迁惨遭帝王之毒刑。

　　后来，司马迁只好隐居山林，继续撰写史书。

　　有一天，司马迁突然感觉小便涩痛不爽，低头一看居然是血尿，他吓坏了。但是司马迁不敢和女儿女婿说，就自己翻阅医籍，从医学书上司马迁得知自己得的是"淋证"（如尿频、尿急、尿短、尿道灼热疼痛等）。

　　这天，他一个人背着竹篓上山采药，在路过一条小溪时，司马迁看到溪流边的石头上长了不少蕨类植物，远看就好像是长在石头表皮上一样。于是他拿出书本一对比，发现这些长在石头上的蕨类植物正是他要寻找的药材。因为古时候人们把鞣制过的皮子称作"韦"，于是"石韦"的名字也就因此而来了。

猜一猜

　　长在石头的皮。（打一植物名）

（答案：石韦）

87

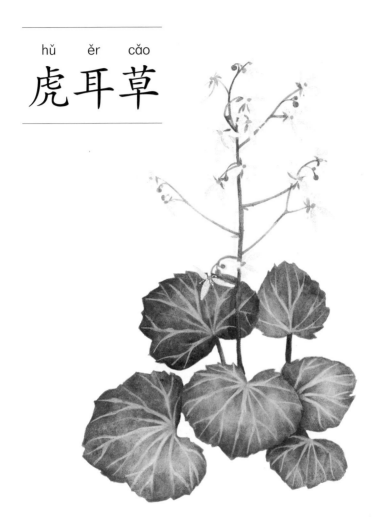

hǔ ěr cǎo

虎耳草

虎耳草的简易养护方法

　　1. 虎耳草喜阴凉、潮湿，要求土壤肥沃、湿润，所以盆栽的话，不能放在太阳底下暴晒。

　　2. 虎耳草繁殖能力很强，可以分株繁殖。将虎耳草浅埋在湿润的腐殖质土壤里，把须根压紧，浇水即可。

别名：石荷叶、金线吊芙蓉、老虎耳
拉丁学名：*Saxifraga stolonifera* Curt.

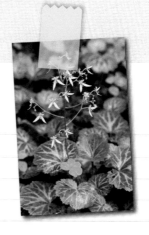

　　虎耳草的故事

　　有一天，一个江湖郎中来到一座山村，当时天气异常闷热，他却看到村里很多人的耳朵都用棉花塞着，有的还往外流脓。郎中觉得奇怪，就向一个年轻人询问。

　　年轻人沮丧地答道："最近村里很多人咳嗽，起疹子，严重的耳朵还流脓，连我 60 多岁的母亲也得了这种病，都被折磨得快不行了。"

　　郎中对年轻人说："我倒有一方，可救你母亲。"

　　年轻人高兴得连忙把郎中带回家中。郎中仔细看了一下年轻人的母亲的耳朵，然后从采药箱里拿出一些叶子圆圆的、开白花的新鲜草药，递给年轻人说："这草药名叫虎耳草，是在你们后山的石崖边上采的，你拿去煎药给你母亲服用，留下一点用来捣汁，滴在她耳朵里。"说完，郎中便起身告辞。

　　年轻人谢过郎中，连忙去煎药捣汁，按照郎中的吩咐给母亲服用。

　　几天下来，年轻人的母亲身上不痒了，耳朵也不流脓了。这位年轻人非常高兴，就奔走着告诉左邻右舍，这件事一下子就传遍了全村。过了一段时间，这种怪病就渐渐消失了，村子里又开始恢复了生机。

猜一猜

　　小小植物岩上生，叶如铜钱，花似长裙。（打一植物名）

（谜底：虎耳草）

89

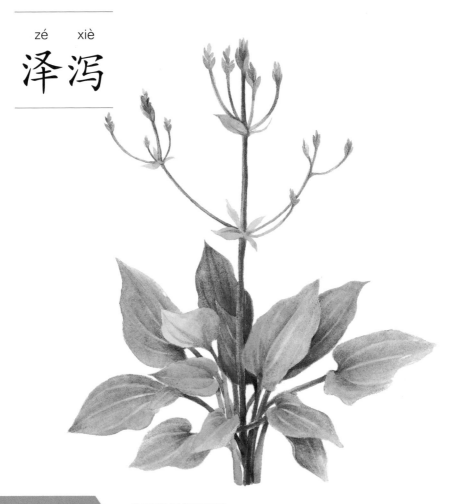

zé xiè
泽泻

你听说过泽泻吗?

别看它名字有些奇怪,其实它是一种价值很高的绿色植物。泽泻除了是利尿良药,还有降血脂的功效。

泽泻中的药物成分在进入人体之后,可以很快地减少人体血液中胆固醇的含量,同时对人体血液中的甘油三酯也有很好的调节作用,因此它可以平衡人体的血脂含量,是预防动脉硬化的天然良药。

别名：水泻、芒芋、鹄泻

拉丁学名：*Alisma plantago-aquatica* L.

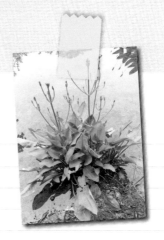

　　　泽泻的故事

　　从前，有一个善良的姑娘，她嫁给了一个老实的农夫泽泻。两人十分恩爱，他们还在屋后的池塘边种了一种开白花的水生植物。

　　哪知，婚后不到半年，泽泻便被抓去当兵。泽泻一走就是三年，音信全无。有一天，一个同村当兵的逃了回来，带来泽泻已战死的噩耗，泽泻的妻子当即昏了过去。这个打击让她本来羸弱的身体更加虚弱了，过了半年，她最终病倒了，小便疼痛，排尿困难，浑身水肿，奄奄一息地躺在床上。

　　泽泻的妻子知道自己快不行了，为了怀念丈夫，她叫邻居二姐到屋后的池塘里挖几棵她和丈夫一起栽的植物煎水给自己喝。二姐含泪点头，照她的吩咐去做。没想到泽泻的妻子喝完汤水后，居然能正常小便，水肿也消失了，身体恢复了正常。

　　泽泻的妻子很惊喜，认为这是她丈夫在保佑她，并且鼓励她好好活下去。她从此振作起来，好好生活。同时，为了纪念自己的丈夫，她把这种神奇的植物叫作"泽泻"，泽泻的名字由此而来。

　　天池洞水。（打一植物名）

（谜底：泽泻）

91

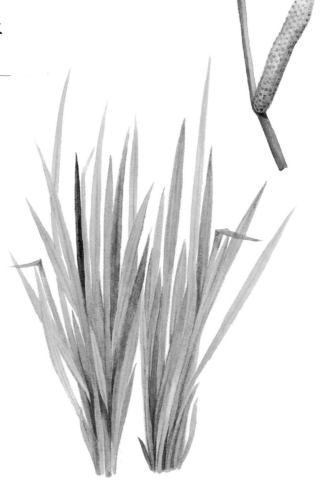

chāng pú

菖蒲

菖蒲在传统节日中的作用

　　民谚说："清明插柳，端午插艾。"端午节，人们除了插艾外，还插菖蒲。家家户户都洒扫庭除，将菖蒲、艾条插于门楣，悬于堂中。那么端午节为什么要挂菖蒲呢？原来，菖蒲的叶子长得像剑，挂在家门口及床头，寓意要斩尽不平之事，全家人都平平安安。

别名：臭蒲、泥菖蒲、香蒲
拉丁学名：*Acorus calamus* L.

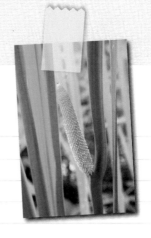

很久以前，有一个妇人，名叫青英，会吟诗作对子，她的丈夫是一个穷秀才。

有一年的五月初四，由于家里一贫如洗，青英就挖了几棵菖蒲，洗净了挂在大门上。她还写了一首诗，贴在大门旁边。

诗是这样写的：

自嫌薄命嫁穷夫，明日端阳祭礼无。

莫叫良辰错过去，聊将清水洗菖蒲。

秀才回家看到这首诗，羞愧难当，就转身离开了。他在路边看到一头老黄牛，便牵了牛想换钱给妻子。可是没走多远，他就被牛主人抓去见知县。

审问之下，秀才一五一十向知县诉说。知县马上派人传秀才青英来。

青英来到公堂上，知县对青英说："既然你会作诗，本县命你再作七绝一首。如成，本县就赏你白银五十两，给你回家去度日。"

青英一听，点头答应。她接过笔墨纸张，想了一会儿，当场就写了这样四句：

滔滔黄水向东流，难洗今朝满面羞。

自笑妾身非织女，郎君何事效牵牛？

知县看完点头表示赞赏，就叫人拿出五十两银子给他们，让他们二人回家了。

青英因家道贫寒，端午节挂菖蒲，竟得到如此好运。此事传开后，每年端午节在大门上挂菖蒲的人家越来越多，就逐渐形成了一种民俗。

四月十四神秘人，九月重阳天南星。（打一植物名）

（谜底：菖蒲）

93

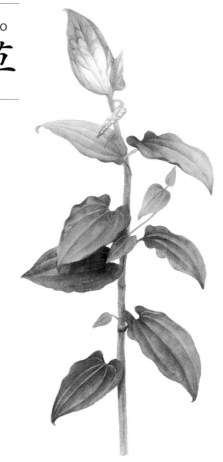

sān bái cǎo

三白草

古代的人如何记录时节？

在古代，没有发达的通讯和记录工具，人们学会了根据植物的生长变化来记录时节。三白草就是其中一种被人们用来记录物候的植物。李时珍的《本草纲目》中写道："三白草，生田泽畔，三月生苗……四月其颠三叶，面上三次变作白色……俗云：一叶白，食小麦；二叶白，食梅杏；三叶白，食黍子。"意思是，三白草的叶子第一次变白时就是麦子成熟的时候；第二次变白时就是梅子和杏子成熟的时候；第三次变白时便可以吃黍子了。

别名：五路叶白、塘边藕、白花莲
拉丁学名：*Saururus chinensis* Baill.

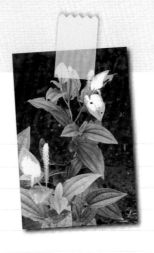

● **三白草的传说**

　　800 多年前，年过花甲的名医刘完素有一次带众弟子上山采药，遇狂风骤雨，回府后即暴病。他不思茶饮，腰酸腿肿，频频如厕，又急又痛，十分痛苦，服了很多药汤均不能奏效，其家人和众弟子惊慌失措。

　　这时，恰逢张元素采药路过，闻之忙入刘府探望，并送上一剂草药。刘完素看那草药像鱼腥草，心想用它能治淋证？犹豫间，有一弟子已拿草药去煎汤，很快便把药煎好了。刘完素一看，药汤略红，气味辛香，才知这药并不是鱼腥草，当即将药汤服下。连服三天，果然病情化险为夷。

　　刘完素忙派人请来张元素当面道谢，并请教所用之妙药为何物。张元素从药筐里取出一束鲜草药，此草药顶生三片叶子为白色。张元素说："此乃三白草，生于塘边泽畔，俗称'塘边藕'，能清热利水，解毒消肿。此为鲜品，跟鱼腥草相似，但鱼腥草气腥臭，阴干后腥气消失；而此药并无腥味。先前送刘先生者为其干品也。"刘完素大开眼界，他将这一种药物的性状、功能、主治等认真记下，并在后来的行医生涯中常常使用，屡见奇效。

猜一猜 ●

　　花开有白叶，说藕不是藕，常在河边有。（打一中药名）

（谜底：三白草）

95

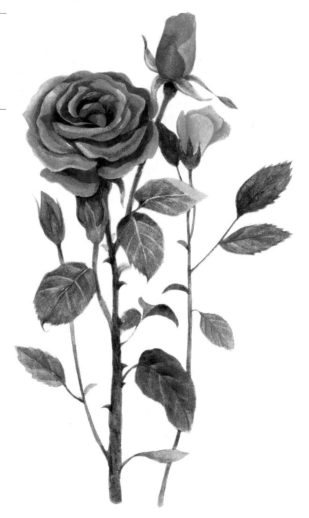

yuè jì

月季

小朋友们，你们知道玫瑰和月季有什么区别吗？

1.茎刺不同。玫瑰：刺硬密，尖细；月季：刺稀疏，扁平。

2.叶子不同。玫瑰：叶凹陷皱缩，无光泽；月季：叶表平展，有光泽。

3.花朵不同。玫瑰：花瓣多开在同一个平面；月季：花瓣不开在同一个平面。

别名：月月红、月月花、四季花
拉丁学名：*Rosa chinensis* Jacq.

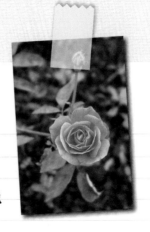

花中皇后——月季花的传说

有一天，王母娘娘过生日，邀请各路仙人来天宫参加宴会。月季花仙子采了满满一篮子月季花，作为献给王母娘娘的寿礼。途中，她看见有一个地方山清水秀，便动了玩心，在山上玩耍起来。

月季花仙子玩了一会儿，才想起贺寿的事，便赶快回到放花篮的地方。"天啊！"她大叫一声，原来那些月季花早已经生根发芽了。她想上前把花拔起来，却被花刺扎了手，只好懊悔地来到天宫。王母娘娘的瑶池里，百花竞相开放。王母娘娘看到月季花仙子，才想起瑶池里独缺月季花。就问月季花仙子："你带来的月季花呢？"月季花仙子慌忙跪下，诉说了刚才发生的事情。王母娘娘大怒，大声喝道："呔！大胆的月季花仙子，玩心太重！来人呀，把她赶出南天门，下凡去吧。"

月季花仙子下凡后，找到了月季花，并且认识了一个勤快的小伙子，月季花仙子对他一见倾心。后来，月季花仙子就嫁给了这个年轻的小伙子。从此，小两口精心培育月季花。经月季花仙子侍弄的月季，开的花格外水灵，什么颜色的都有。因为月季花月月开，人们都非常喜爱，所以月季花逐渐遍布全国。

每个月的最后一天。（打一植物名）

（谜底：月季。月季，俗称"月月红"，可理解为"月尽"。）

lián

莲

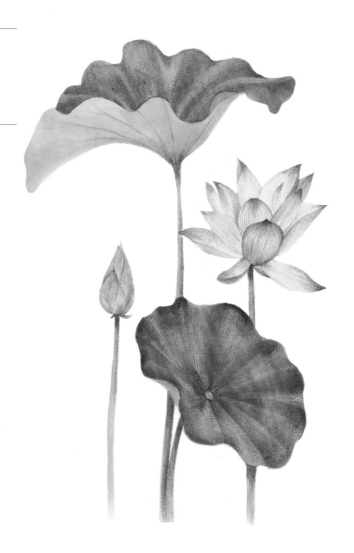

莲的知识

　　莲又称为"荷"。莲全身皆宝，藕和莲子能食用；莲子、藕、藕节、叶、花及莲心等都可入药。莲在我国有着悠久的栽培和食用历史，我国是世界上栽培莲最多的国家。

别名：芙蓉、莲藕、荷花
拉丁学名：*Nelumbo nucifera* Gaertn.

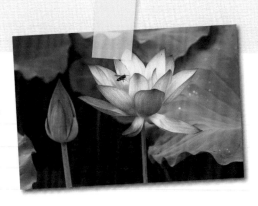

草药小故事　　**荷花的传说**

很久以前，浚河一带人烟稀少。有一个姓张的大伯，以打鱼为生，他没有老伴，因此收养了一个儿子，这个儿子一岁大。

有一天，张大伯又来打鱼，忽见河水中冒出一个竹筒来，里面传出小孩的哭声。张大伯忙把竹筒捞上来，小心地凿开，只见里面有一个很小的女婴，非常可爱，张大伯甚是喜欢，便收养了她。

不知不觉地，两个孩子长大了。到了十七八岁，哥哥长得英俊，妹妹长得水灵。特别是妹妹，粉红的小脸蛋如出水的荷花，就像仙女下凡般漂亮。

没有人知道这女婴就是荷花仙子，因为她做错了事，被玉皇大帝罚到人间。

有一天半夜，天兵天将下来催促荷花仙子回天宫，手里还拿着兵器。荷花仙子心念张大伯的养育之恩，不觉泪流满面，泪水滴到水里，随即长出一片荷花来。她咬破手指，在手绢上写下几个字，抛下手绢后就随天兵天将离去了。

天亮后，张大伯起床后不见女儿，忙到门外去找，只见清池里长满了荷花，池边放着一块手绢。张大伯找人一念，才知道女儿是荷花仙子下凡。荷花仙子说，养育之恩日后必相报，张大伯如果想念她，就到门前看看荷花，那是她的化身。

猜一猜

远看像把小绿伞，近看像个大绿盘，水珠掉进绿盘里，好像珍珠滚滚掉。（打一花名）

（谜底：荷花）

补骨脂

bǔ gǔ zhī

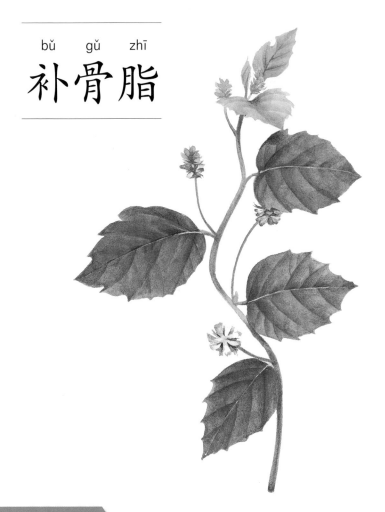

补骨脂有毒，为什么还可以做药？

人们常说："是药三分毒。"补骨脂也有毒，但是它确实是很好的补阳药，在使用它时要遵循医嘱。补骨脂还是治疗白癜风的良药，使用过程中为避免出现对人体不利的毒副作用，要配合日光或长波紫外线照射治疗。同时，应注意眼睛防护，免受紫外线损伤，最好于傍晚服药，服药后 24 小时内戴防紫外线护目镜。

别名：破故纸、和兰苋、胡韭子
拉丁学名：*Cullen corylifolium* Medik.

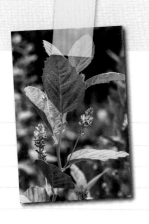

补骨脂的传说

相传，唐朝元和年间，75 岁高龄的相国郑愚被皇上任命为海南节度使。年迈体衰的郑愚只好马不停蹄地前去赴任。无奈路途遥远，旅途劳顿和水土不服使他筋疲力尽，浑身有气无力，一副快要断气的样子。性命都难保，更别说料理政务了。为了给他治病，随从给他请了很多大夫。郑愚服用了很多方剂，始终不见效。

听闻此事，诃陵国李氏三番登府推荐中药补骨脂。郑愚抱着试试看的心理，按照李氏介绍的方法服药。服后七八日，他渐觉有效，又连服十日，原先的那些浑身无力的症状都消失了。

后来，郑愚常服用此药，到 82 岁辞官回京时，身体还十分硬朗，于是他将此药广为介绍，并吟诗一首："七年使节向边隅，人言方知药物殊。奇得春光采在手，青娥休笑白髭须。"

从此，补骨脂因其温肾助阳的作用而广为人知。

猜一猜

尘封的旧人来信。（打一中药名）

（谜底：补骨脂，即故旧的纸信。）

植物果实绘画技巧

为了感谢手绘爱好者们的支持，本书特别增加手绘小课堂，邀请人气插画师乐毛线为大家详细讲解药用植物栝楼的绘画过程。还等什么，拿起笔来跟乐毛线一起画出漂亮的药用植物吧！

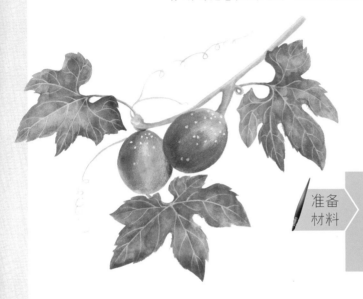

准备材料

60 色水溶彩色色铅笔
固体水彩
水彩画笔
300 g 细纹水彩纸

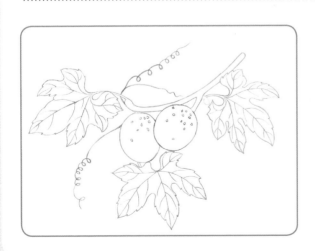

1. 将彩色铅笔削尖，轻轻地画出栝楼的整体造型，在用线时可适当注意线的变化。栝楼的果实圆润饱满，打型的时候可以用一个圆圈确定，接着画出不同角度的叶子。

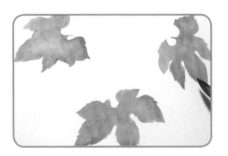

2. 接着，简单地用草绿色固体水彩画出叶片基础色，混合深绿色勾画边缘叶子的暗面转折，保持下笔的干净利落，切勿重复叠色。

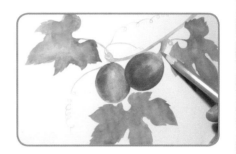

4. 接下来换上水溶彩色铅笔开始第二轮的上色，以加深主体细节，明确光影关系。以强化栝楼整体体积为目的，加深藤蔓的暗部。

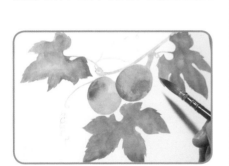

3. 用橘黄色固体水彩为栝楼的果实铺上底色，注意投影以及暗面的深浅过度。受光的影响，受光处颜色偏浅，背光处颜色较深并伴着偏绿的环境色，紧接着勾勒栝楼的枝藤。

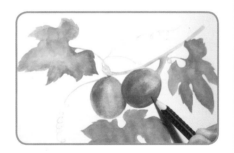

5. 用橘红色彩色铅笔加深果实的明暗交界线，用棕色彩色铅笔描绘果实与果实之间的投影，用橘黄色铅笔加强果实的过渡面以及更换不同的彩色铅笔调整藤蔓的色彩层次。始终以中间的橘黄色果实为视觉中心。

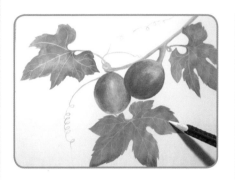

6. 由中间向外慢慢刻画，注意观察栝楼叶子的叶脉走向并使用白色彩色铅笔勾勒出来。上色的时候注意植物的远近关系，离视线近的地方细节更丰富。

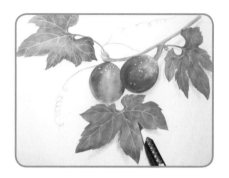

8. 叶子转折边缘的色彩变化，通过刻画这些小细节，让画面更有层次。

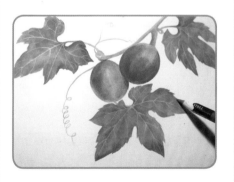

7. 最后描绘栝楼的叶片细节，由于受到光的影响，注意叶子从边缘处向内由深变浅的颜色变化。

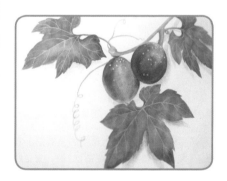

9. 最后用银色彩色铅笔和灰色彩色铅笔为栝楼添加投影，让叶片及果实跃然纸上。

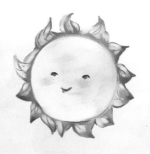

Hello, my friends!
Welcome to the world of Chinese herbal medicines.
Are you ready to get to know them?

Gou Wen

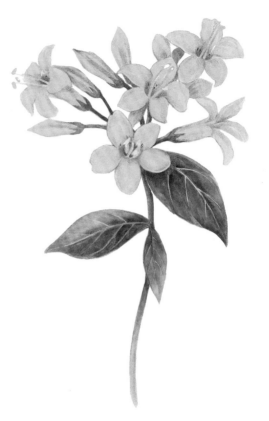

Kids! How much do you know about the Duan Chang Cao in ancient times?

It is mentioned by Li Shizhen (a famous doctor in ancient China) in the *Compendium of Materia Medica* and refers to the Chinese herb Gou Wen (*Gelsemium elegans*). Its toxin has significant analgesic and hypnotic effects.

In ancient times, herbs that caused severe toxic reactions in the gastrointestinal tract after ingestion were often referred to as Duan Chang Cao. Herbs such as *Aconitum carmichaelii* in the Ranunculaceae family, *Stellera chamaejasme* in the Thymelaeaceae family, and *Euphorbia pekinensis* in the Euphorbiaceae family were given the name due to their pronounced toxicity. Consuming these Duan Chang Cao could lead to fatal consequences.

Chinese Common Names: Heartbreak Grass, Da Cha Yao (tea-shaped plant), Hu Man Teng

Latin Name: *Gelsemium elegans* Benth.

Duan Chang Cao and Emperor Qianlong

During the Qing Dynasty (1616-1911 AD), Emperor Qianlong put on casual clothes and went to Zhenjiang (a city of Jiangsu Province, China) to personally investigate. After staying at an inn, he felt an unusual itch and decided to buy medicine in an herbal medicine shop.

"Forgive my late-night disturbance, I want to buy some herbs," after knocking on the door, the young and refined Emperor bowed to the herbalist with the grace of an affluent gentleman.

"Please have a seat, I haven't retired to bed yet," the middle-aged herbalist replied as he opened the door.

Emperor Qianlong explained his symptoms to the herbalist. After a careful examination, the herbalist said, "You are suffering from a skin disease called 'scabies', which is treatable but requires strict adherence to medical advice. After applying the medicine, you should avoid scratching directly with your hands, and more importantly, you can not take it orally as this herb is highly toxic."

"Could you tell me the name of this herb?" Emperor Qianlong curiously inquired.

"It's called Duan Chang Cao. Legend has it that when Shennong (an ancient Chinese Emperor who discovered herbal medicines) tasted a variety of herbs, he encountered a vine with its leaves growing opposite each other, bearing pale yellow flowers. He picked a few tender leaves and tasted them. Yet upon chewing and swallowing, the toxicity was unleashed, causing severe damage to his intestines. This vine is now known as Duan Chang Cao," the herbalist replied.

Shortly after, Emperor Qianlong's skin disease was cured. He generously rewarded the herbalist and wrote the words "Shennong Bai Cao Tang" (Shennong's Hall of Hundred Herbs) for herbalist's medicine shop, which made the herbal medicine shop renowned around the world.

Bi Ma

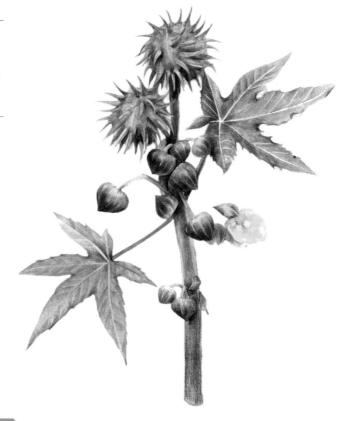

Kids! Do you know how to sow Bi Ma?

Before sowing, you need to soak the bean seeds of Bi Ma in water at a temperature of 40-50°C for 24 hours, then remove them and bury them in moist sand. The seeds generally take 5-7 days to germinate. Once they sprout, you can sow them immediately.

For seeds that have been stored for some time, you can soak them in water at a temperature of 40-50°C for 48 hours to soften the hard shell and allow the seeds to absorb enough water, thus accelerating the germination process. Once some of the Bi Ma seeds have sprouted, it's time to sow them.

Chinese Common Names: Da Ma Zi, Lao Ma Zi, Cao Ma

Latin Name: *Ricinus communis* L.

Jonah and Bi Ma

During the time of Jeroboam II (790-750 BC), Israelis in the Assyrian kingdom received blessings and guidance from God but refused to serve him. As a result, God sent a prophet named Jonah to warn them: due to their sins, the city of Nineveh in the Assyrian kingdom would be destroyed within 40 days.

Upon receiving the warning, the people of Nineveh began to pray to God. God listened to their prayers and decided not to destroy the city.

Yet Jonah disagreed and sucked, ignoring the God. He constructed a small shelter on a place where he could overlook and observe the city. However, nothing happened except for the scorching sun beating down on him.

God transplanted a Bi Ma to provide shade for Jonah, making him feel much cooler.

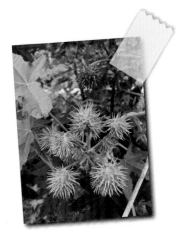

However, the next day, it withered because God sent a worm to bite its roots. The plant that shaded him from the sun died, while the wicked city of Nineveh remained unharmed, which provoked his wrath.

Then, God warned Jonah, "You care about the Bi Ma even though you don't plant or nurture it. How could I not have compassion for all the people and the plants in the city of Nineveh?"

Upon hearing this, Jonah finally realized God's kind intention.

Ji Ying Su

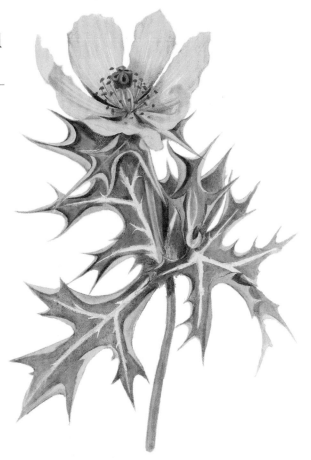

Where are Ji Ying Su's seeds?

As the end of summer approaches, the fruits of Ji Ying Su mature. Harvest the fruits, dry them, and crush them to remove their husks. Then, we will get their seeds.

The seeds of the plant are toxic, so don't consume them accidentally, as it may lead to diarrhea.

Chinese Common Names: Ci Ying Su (Mexican Prickly Poppy; "Ci" means thorn; it has thorns on its leaves and stems), Lao Shu Ji (its leaves resemble the wings of a bat, which were referred to as mice in ancient times)

Latin Name: *Argemone mexicana* L.

The Story of Ji Ying Su

In Greek mythology, Demeter is the goddess of the harvest and agriculture, as well as the mother of the gods. Demeter and the supreme ruler of the universe, Zeus, had a lovely daughter named Persephone.

Due to Demeter's good management in agriculture, the world was always blessed with warm weather and abundant crops.

One day, when Persephone was picking flowers, the earth suddenly split up. Then, Hades who was the ruler of the Underworld emerged, kidnapping her and forcibly making her his queen. Upon learning that Hades had taken Persephone, Demeter felt devastated and used the juice of Ji Ying Su for alleviating her pain and sorrow.

As Demeter lost her daughter, she had no interest in managing agriculture. Consequently, the land became barren; humanity faced the threat of death; and the gods were deprived of their offerings. Zeus, the supreme god, ordered Hades to return Persephone. However, Hades compelled Persephone to eat a pomegranate seed from the Underworld, binding her to spend only 1/4 of the time on Earth with her mother, while the rest was in the Underworld.

Demeter rejoiced when Persephone returned to the Earth, bringing warm days of spring when flowers blossom and the recovery of all living things. However, when Persephone left her mother to return to the Underworld, Demeter was shrouded in sorrow, leading to the withering of all living things and the changing seasons throughout the year.

Shang Lu

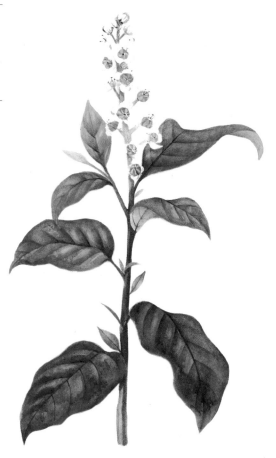

Can Shang Lu also make rouge?

Shang Lu, also known as "Yan Zhi Cao". When the round and flat berries of Shang Lu ripen, they turn deep red-purple or black, resembling miniature grapes. In folk traditions, people often use it as a rouge applied to girls' foreheads, therefore it has its nickname "Yan Zhi Cao". There is an ancient saying, "Yan Zhi Cao: woman's heart".

The fruit of Shang Lu has a bright color and juicy taste, appearing to be delicious. However, it is poisonous, and children should never eat it.

Chinese Common Names: Shan Luo Bo, Jian Zhong Xiao, Ye Hu

Latin Name: *Phytolacca acinosa* Roxb.

The Story of Shang Lu

During the Kaiyuan Era (713-741 AD) of Emperor Xuanzong in the Tang Dynasty, there was a village named Daowan on the edge of the Southern Mountain. In this village, a quack named Shi Fu picked up some medical skills from others and combined them with his persuasive tongue, transforming himself into a "divine healer".

As time went on, people from the surrounding villages stopped seeking medical help from him. Shi Fu then slung his medicine cabinet and swaggered onto the road, waving a banner writing "Ji Shi Huo Fo, Miao Shou Hui Chun", which meant that he had such excellent medical skills that he could bring a patient back to life.

Shi Fu came to a desolate mountain covered with countless graves. At that moment, a woodcutter carrying firewood descended from the mountain. Due to his haste, the woodcutter accidentally knocked Shi Fu unconscious.

Thinking he had killed Shi Fu, the woodcutter got scared and ran away as fast as he could.

When Shi Fu regained consciousness, the sun had already set. He seemed to hear the cries coming from the lush grass near the graves. He discovered a fleshy, inverted cone-shaped plant. Mistaking it for ginseng due to its resemblance to radish and its root similar to ginseng, Shi Fu bit it immediately. However, he soon experienced nausea, vomiting, abdominal pain, and severe diarrhea. He felt distressed and sought out a doctor. Knowing what happened to Shi Fu, the doctor consulted medical books and finally remove the toxins.

From that day on, Shi Fu dedicated himself to studying medical books and refrained from haphazardly treating people. The ginseng he dug up that night was named Ye Hu by Shi Fu because of the sounds it emitted that night.

Ye Gan

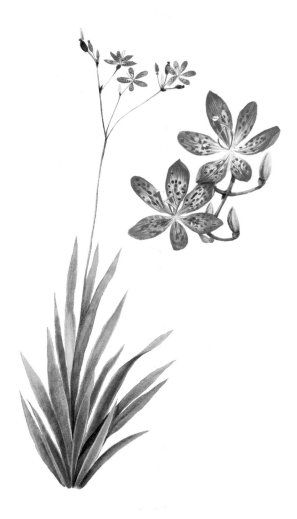

As Ye Gan and iris are very similar in appearance, how to identify them?

1. Ye Gan: (1) The dried rhizome is irregularly nodular; (2) The surface exhibits yellow-brown or black-brown spots; (3) It has a bitter taste.

2. Iris: (1) The dried rhizome is flat and cylindrical; (2) The surface appears gray-brown; (3) It has a slightly bitter taste with a hint of pungency.

Chinese Common Names: Ye Xuan Hua, Jiao Jian Cao, Bian Zhu

Latin Name: *Belamcanda chinensis* Redouté.

The Story of Ye Gan

Long ago, there was a woodcutter living at the foot of Mao'er Mountain, making a living by chopping wood. He lived a difficult life as he had to take care of his blind mother.

One summer, the woodcutter caught a cold with a sore throat and hadn't been able to go up the mountain to chop wood for several days. With no money, he could only borrow a bowl of rice from a neighbor to cook porridge for his mother.

After his mother finished eating, the weak woodcutter dragged himself up the mountain to chop wood. Due to his physical weakness and lack of food, he fainted by a stream.

When the woodcutter woke up, he found himself lying amidst a profusion of flowers, which resembled butterflies around him. Due to extreme hunger, the woodcutter couldn't help eating the flowering plant. Although it tasted bitter at first, there was sweet afterward and a refreshing feeling in his throat. Before long, the woodcutter's throat got better and he felt more energetic than before.

At this moment, a beautiful and kind deity appeared beside the woodcutter, telling him that the flower he ate was called Ye Gan which could treat throat pain.

Worried about his elderly mother at home, the woodcutter expressed his gratitude to the deity and rushed back home. Touched by his filial piety, the deity gifted him many seeds of Ye Gan and explained how to grow them.

Upon returning home, the woodcutter followed the deity's instructions and planted numerous medicinal herbs near his house. He generously taught the villagers how to plant these herbs without reservation.

From then on, the woodcutter and the villagers lived a worry-free life by cultivating these medicinal herbs.

Ru Qie

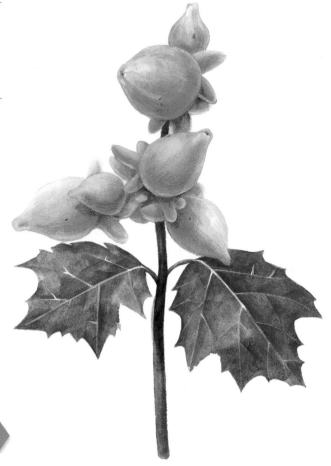

Toxic Fruit with Golden Luster — Ru Qie

Ru Qie is the latest hit among potted flowers, named for its fruit shape resembling breasts. Its fruit remains unchanged with a golden luster for long, symbolizing prosperity, generations living together, and good fortune. It also conveys the meaning of Wu Zi Deng Ke (It symbolizes prosperity for the family and illustrious achievements for the descendants). These reasons make it a popular flower for Chinese New Year. However, Ru Qie is toxic and should not be consumed raw; otherwise, it can cause harm to the body.

Chinese Common Names: Wu Zhi Qie, Wu Jiao Ding Qie, Wu Zi Deng Ke

Latin Name: *Solanum mammosum* L.

A Tale of Wu Jiao Ding Qie

In the mysterious ancient times, there was a village inhabited by Indian in the beautiful Americas. In this village, there were two brothers. The younger brother was frail since childhood and the elder brother wholeheartedly took care of his younger sibling. Every day, the elder brother went hunting in the forest while the younger brother gathered fruits near the village.

One day, in his eagerness to chase prey, the elder brother accidentally tumbled into a ditch. He injured his foot during the fall and also bumped into a large tree, losing his consciousness. Due to the dampness in the forest, his wounds became infected.

The younger brother leaned against the door, waiting for his brother, and eventually fell asleep. In his dream, a tree deity communicated with him, revealing the condition of his elder brother. The younger brother felt terrified and asked the tree deity where to find his brother. The tree deity guided the younger brother down a small path and instructed him, "Near me, there is a grass with short soft hairs and flat prickles on the stems, bearing five-angular golden fruits. Bring the small golden fruits back, dry them, and apply them to the wounds to alleviate the swelling on your brother."

Upon waking up, the younger brother immediately followed the path indicated by the tree deity to find his brother and helped him back home. He also found the small golden fruits near the big tree, gathered some, and followed the tree deity's instructions to treat his brother's injuries. Soon, the elder brother recovered.

Later, the two brothers expressed their respect and gratitude to the tree deity and named the tiny golden fruits "Wu Jiao Ding Qie".

Yang Jin Hua

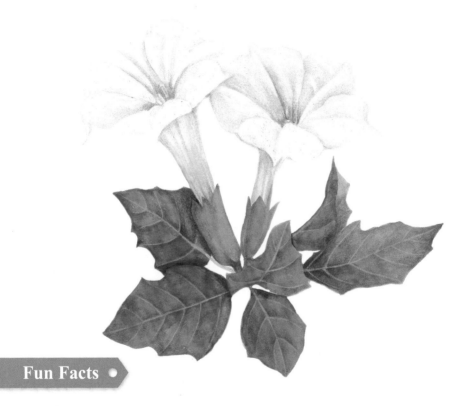

Traditional Anesthetic — Ma Fei San

It was said that around the year 200 AD, the renowned Chinese physician Hua Tuo used Ma Fei San as an anesthetic for patients undergoing bone scraping and abdominal surgery (This tale appears to contradict scientific knowledge and lacks archaeological evidence to support it).

Ma Fei San is a traditional Chinese medicine anesthetic made from Yang Jin Hua.

Chinese Common Names: Bai Hua Man Tuo Luo, Nao Yang Hua, Chou Ma Zi Hua

Latin Name: *Datura metel* L.

The First Anesthetic — Ma Fei San

According to legend, one day, Hua Tuo encountered a peculiar patient: he had tightly clenched teeth with foaming at the mouth, clenched fists, and lay motionless on the ground. Hua Tuo approached, observed the patient's condition, checked the pulse, and felt the forehead, finding everything to be normal. Hua Tuo then inquired about the patient's medical history, and the family replied, "He was very healthy and strong without any illness. However, today he accidentally consumed several Chou Ma Zi Hua, which led to these symptoms."

Hua Tuo promptly requested them to bring Chou Ma Zi Hua. The patient's family presented it with its flowers and fruits to Hua Tuo. Hua Tuo sniffed, examined it, and even tasted the petal, immediately feeling dizzy and numbness in his mouth.

By clearing away heat and toxic material, Hua Tuo successfully cured the patient. Before leaving, he asked for nothing in return except for a bundle of the plant with its flowers and fruits.

From that day, Hua Tuo began conducting experiments with the plant. He tasted the leaves, then the flowers, and finally the fruits and roots. The results of his experiments showed that the fruit of Chou Ma Zi Hua had excellent anesthetic effects. Hua Tuo visited many doctors and gathered some medicines with anesthetic properties. After numerous formulations, he finally succeeded in creating an anesthetic. Then he combined the anesthetic with hot wine, improving its effectiveness.

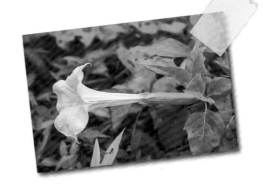

Hua Tuo gave the formulated anesthetic a name — Ma Fei San.

Ding Xiang Luo Le

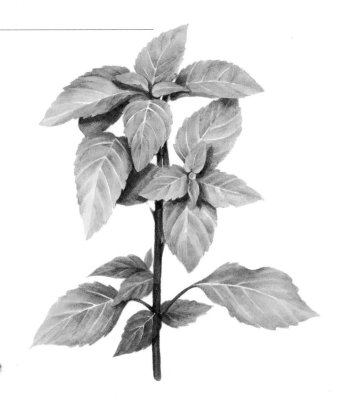

The essential oil of Luo Le has various uses

1. It is beneficial for the respiratory system. It can be used to treat cold and cough symptoms, and assist in relieving asthma, bronchitis, nasal mucosa inflammation and indigestion.

2. It can uplift the spirit and heighten sensitivity; it has a calming effect on symptoms of hysteria and can soothe depression and alleviate headaches.

3. It can tighten the skin, balance oil secretion; it has a slight stimulating effect on sensitive skin.

Chinese Common Name: Chou Cao
Latin Name: *Ocimum gratissimum* L.

The Legend of Ding Xiang Luo Le

Long ago, there was a beautiful girl who fell in love with a handsome young man. The young man came from a destitute family. There lived a wealthy man in the town who had been captivated by the girl's beauty and had proposed to her multiple times, all of which were rejected by the girl. The girl's family, however, were determined to have her marry the wealthy man to improve their living conditions.

The girl's two brothers harbored a deep hatred for the young man, believing that he had shattered their dreams of living a prosperous life. The brothers repeatedly set traps, intentionally framing and scheming against the young man in an attempt to make the girl give up him. However, their conspiracies were exposed each time, and the girl ultimately chose to be with the young man. Their relationship became more resilient.

To make her brothers give up, the girl decided to officially engage with the young man on the Qixi Festival (Chinese Valentine's Day). Upon learning this, her two brothers were on the verge of collapse and decided to kill the young man.

Finally, one day, the two brothers deceived the young man into a desolate wilderness and murdered him. Upon discovering this, the girl was heartbroken and cried for seven days and seven nights. In the very place where the young man was killed, she planted a Ding Xiang Luo Le.

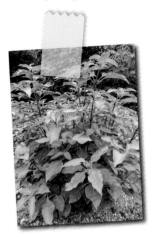

The following year, Luo Le emitted a fragrance of Ding Xiang (cloves). Since then, this plant has been known for its intoxicating aroma like Ding Xiang. And that is why the plant was named Ding Xiang Luo Le.

Zi Su

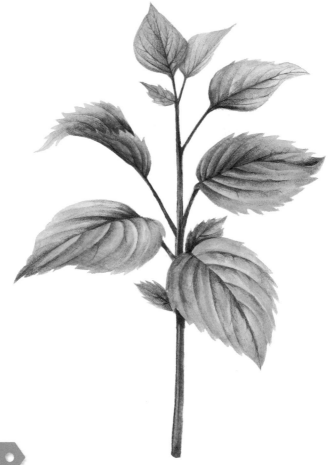

Zi Su has multiple uses in our daily lives

Zi Su has significant uses in our daily lives. It can be used as a spice and a side dish, and it is also effective in neutralizing the toxicity of seafood such as shrimp and crab. Additionally, it can be used to treat colds. In summer, if one has a cold with symptoms like chills, fever, cough, asthma, and some intestinal disorders, he could drink the soup made from Zi Su's leaves or consum the young leaves raw, which confirmed quite effective.

Chinese Common Names: Chi Su, Hong Su, Hong Zi Su
Latin Name: *Perilla frutescens* Britt.

The Legend of Zi Su

According to legend, on the Double Ninth Festival, namely on the ninth day of the ninth lunar month, Hua Tuo took his students to the town. On the way, they suddenly saw an otter catch and swallow a large fish, which made itself so uncomfortable that it rolled and tossed on the shore. Later, the otter crawled to a patch of purple grass by the shore, ate some purple plants, circled a few times, and soon, it comfortably swam away.

Upon reaching the town, they drank in a tavern. Nearby, some young men were competing to eat crabs. Hua Tuo thought that crabs were cold in nature and that eating too many could lead to illness, so he persuaded them to stop politely. However, the young men ignored Hua Tuo's good advice. One of them even sarcastically said, "Old man, are you craving some? I'll break off a piece for you to taste."

Hua Tuo sighed and had to sit down to enjoy his drink.

Little did they know that after two hours, all the young men suddenly suffered from stomachaches. Some were in such pain that beads of sweat appeared on their foreheads, screaming in pain, others rolled on the ground clutching their stomachs.

Sitting near those men, Hua Tuo instructed his students to gather some purple plants from the lowland outside the tavern and give them to the young men. Shortly after consuming the plants, their stomachaches eased. Therefore, they repeatedly thanked Hua Tuo. Upon returning home, they spread the word about how skilled Hua Tuo was in the art of medicine.

Because this medicinal herb is purple and brings comfort when being ingested, Hua Tuo named it Zi Shu ("Zi" means purple and "Shu" means comfort). Later, due to its similar pronunciation, people started calling it Zi Su.

Hui Xiang

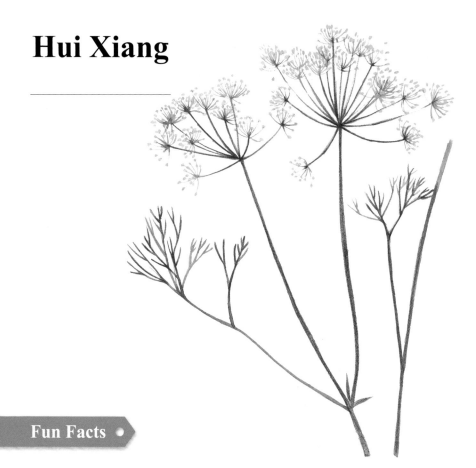

Is Hui Xiang (Fennel) the same as cumin seeds?

Many readers have come across both cumin seeds and Xiao Hui Xiang in their daily lives, but are they the same thing? We don't believe many readers know that, let's take a look at the differences between them.

Although they are both spices with similar shapes, their flavors are different. Hui Xiang has slightly larger seeds, and they are somewhat plump with a greenish color, while cumin seeds are somewhat elongated with a yellowish color. Can you distinguish between them now?

Chinese Common Names: Xiao Hui Xiang, Tu Hui Xiang
Latin Name: *Foeniculum vulgare* Mill.

The Story about a Rich Merchant and Xiao Hui Xiang

In the late Qing Dynasty (1616-1911 AD), a Russian merchant named Mikhaylov came to China. Having heard about Emperor Qianlong's fascination with the picturesque landscapes of Jiangnan, he also wanted to appreciate the beauty of the region. One day, he set out and took a boat trip to West Lake in Hangzhou. While he was enjoying the stunning scenery, he was suddenly struck by a severe colic attack. The pain was so intense that he clutched his stomach and screamed in agony, rolling on the ground. The Russian doctors accompanying him were panicked when watching Mikhaylov being tormented by the illness, but they were helpless. At this urgent moment, a boatman saw what happened and quickly recommended an old Chinese doctor to them.

At this critical juncture, the Russian doctors had no choice but to let the old Chinese doctor take charge. The old chinese doctor calmly took out 1 liang (equivalent to 50 g) Chinese medicine, Xiao Hui Xiang, ground it into coarse powder, and instructed Mikhaylov to take it with 2 liang (equivalent to 100 g) of Shaoxing yellow wine from Zhejiang Province. Approximately 20 minutes later, Mikhaylov's colic pain miraculously relieved and quickly disappeared. The accompanying Russian doctors were astonished that these small seeds could cure the sudden and strange illness. They all sought the secret from the old Chinese doctor, who generously told them that it was the seeds of Xiao Hui Xiang.

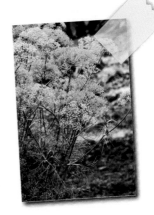

Upon learning that his pain had been cured by Xiao Hui Xiang, Mikhaylov exclaimed in amazement. At the same time, he deeply admired the wonders of traditional Chinese medicine. Then the story has become known to all.

Jiang Huang

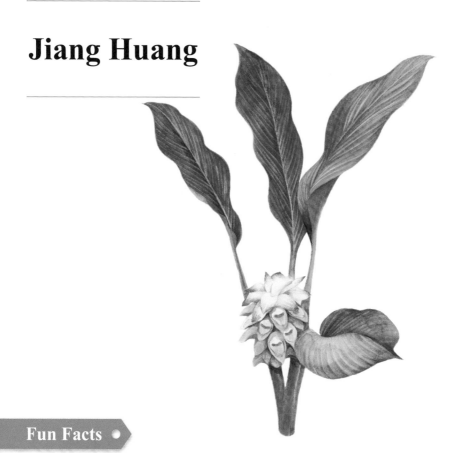

Apart from being used as medicine, what other purposes does Jiang Huang serve?

Let's explore some other uses of Jiang Huang in our daily lives. It belongs to the ginger plant family and is often added to food as a spice. Jiang Huang powder (Turmeric powder) is the most common form. It is an orange-yellow powder made by grinding the boiled and dried rhizomes of the plant. This powder serves as a food additive and is an essential component of curry powder. Additionally, Jiang Huang is used in Pao Cai (Chinese pickled vegetables).

Chinese Common Names: Bao Ding Xiang, Huang Jiang, Yu Jin
Latin Name: *Curcuma longa* L.

The Story of Jiang Huang

According to legend, a long time ago, the Han River and its tributary Tianhe River experienced three consecutive years of severe drought, resulting in a complete failure of crops. Even the owner of a restaurant in the town nearby, who had been operating for years, went out to escape the famine, leaving only the cook to watch over the restaurant. The cook was called as "Army Cook" by the locals because he was diligent in his work and kind to others.

One evening, a beggar with a limp appeared in front of the restaurant, and "Army Cook" generously gave him the only bowl of sweet potato porridge. When the cook asked about his home, the old beggar replied that he lived at the Tianhe Mountain. With these words, the old beggar disappeared.

The cook was concerned about him and decided to go up the mountain to find him the next day. By noon, exhausted and hungry, he collapsed by the roadside. In a daze, he saw an old man bowing his head on the hillside, digging a root with hairs and placing it in a pot to steam. Upon closer inspection, "Army Cook" realized that it was the old man who appeared in the restaurant last night. Just as the cook was about to approach the old man, he woke up abruptly. When "Army Cook" regained consciousness, he found himself lying on a dense bed of Jiang Huang (turmeric). Feeling rejuvenated, he dug out many hairy roots along the stems and leaves.

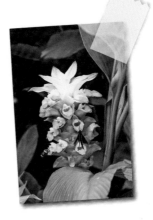

Bringing these roots back home, "Army Cook" steamed and cooked them according to the method shown by the old man in his dream. Once being peeled and cooked, the roots turned out to be delicious and fragrant. Those who tried it found it tasty and filling. The story quickly spread along the banks of the Tianhe River and became well-known to all.

Yi Zhi

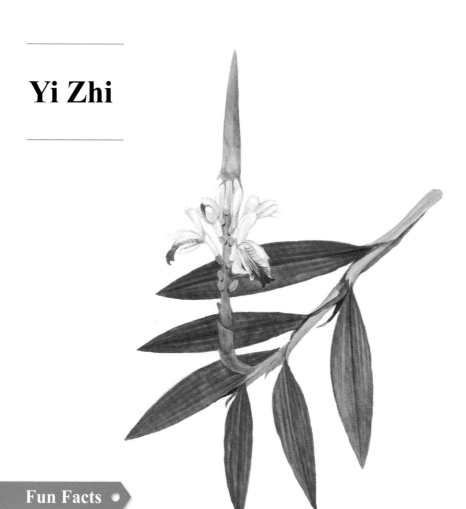

Yi Zhi and ginger look very similar, so how do we distinguish between them?

Firstly, from the perspective of medicinal parts, ginger uses its rhizomes, while Yi Zhi uses its fruits which are harvested when they turn red at the turn of summer and autumn. Secondly, ginger has irregular shaped rhizomes, while Yi Zhi's fruits are oval in shape with slightly pointed ends, featuring longitudinally uneven raised ridges and special aroma.

Chinese Common Names: Yi Zhi Zi, Yi Zhi Ren, Zhai Ding Zi
Latin Name: *Alpinia oxyphylla* Miq.

The Legend of Yi Zhi Ren

Legend has it that a long time ago, there was a wealthy man, who in his later years, finally had a son and named him Laifu which meant lucky arrival. Laifu was frail and sickly since childhood with an exceptionally large head. He often drooled and was dull and sluggish. Additionally, he wet the bed every day. As years passed, Laifu remained quiet and had a very poor memory. At the age of ten, he still couldn't count, often forget the previous numbers while counting on. Despite the wealthy man seeking renowned doctors in the vicinity, Laifu's illnesses remained incurable.

One day, a Taoist happened to travel there. After hearing the wealthy man's description of his son's condition, the Taoist told him, "Eight thousand miles away from here, there is a magical fruit that can cure your son's illness." The Taoist drew a picture on the ground, depicting a small tree with leaves resembling ginger leaves and several olive-shaped fruits at the roots. After completing the drawing, the Taoist departed.

Determined to find the magical fruit himself, the wealthy man embarked on a difficult journey. After overcoming numerous hardships, he finally found the tree, then plucked a full bag of fruits and returned.

After consuming the magical fruit, Laifu became cheerful, intelligent, and adorable, appearing to be a completely different person. At the age of 18, he participated in the imperial civil examination and was the top scorer. In commemoration of the magical fruit that changed Laifu's destiny, people named it the "Champion Fruit". Due to its cognitive-enhancing property that makes people smarter, it was also called "Yi Zhi Ren", which means wisdom-enhancing in Chinese.

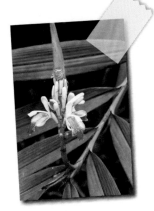

Huo Xiang

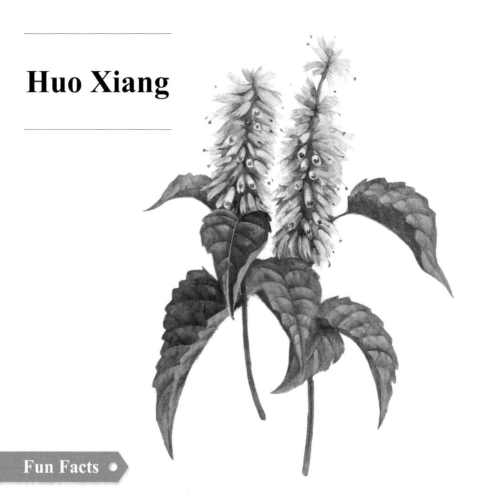

Besides being used to create Huo Xiang Zheng Qi Shui (a liquid herbal formula), Huo Xiang has other benefits

1. In terms of landscaping, green belts of Huo Xiang are often used for mass planting along flower paths, pond edges, and courtyard areas.

2. In terms of nutrition, Huo Xiang has a high of calcium and carotene. The whole plant contains aromatic essential oils, which have a certain inhibitory effect on various pathogenic fungi. Aromatic essential oils are also used as raw materials in various traditional Chinese medicines.

Chinese Common Names: He Xiang, Ye Huo Xiang, Su Huo Xiang
Latin Name: *Agastache rugosa* O. Ktze.

The Legend of Huo Xiang

Long ago, in the deep mountains, there lived a family with a brother and sister named Huo Xiang. They depended on each other. After the brother got married, he joined the military, leaving only his wife and his sister to take care of each other.

One summer, the sister-in-law suffered from heatstroke due to overwork and suddenly developed a high fever, chills, headache, nausea, and fatigue. Huo Xiang quickly helped her onto the bed and determined to venture deep into the mountains to gather medicinal herbs to cure her sister-in-law.

Huo Xiang was out for an entire day and returned when it was dark. She carried a small basket of herbs in her hands with her eyes staring blankly. As soon as she entered the house, she collapsed to the ground. The sister-in-law quickly got out of bed to support her and asked what happened to her. Then the sister-in-law realized that Huo Xiang had been bitten by a venomous snake while collecting herbs. As the sister-in-law exclaimed in shock, she lifted Huo Xiang's right foot, preparing to suck the venom out the bite. However, Huo Xiang adamantly refused, fearing that the sister-in-law might get poisoned. It was already too late when the villagers heard the sister-in-law's cry for help and brought a doctor.

Using the herbs collected by Huo Xiang, the sister-in-law managed to cure her illness. With the help of the villagers, she buried Huo Xiang. In memory of Huo Xiang's sacrifice, the sister-in-law affectionately named the fragrant herb "Huo Xiang" and encouraged everyone to plant it around their homes and along the roadsides to make it more accessible. From then on, the reputation of the herb "Huo Xiang" spread far and wide, successfully treating many patients suffering from heatstroke.

In the later years, because "Huo Xiang" was herb, people added "Cao" (艹) character (it is a basic structural part of Chinese characters, generally, it is related to plants) on the "Huo" (霍) character (generally, it refers to a surname), writing it as "Huo Xiang" (藿香).

Ning Meng Cao

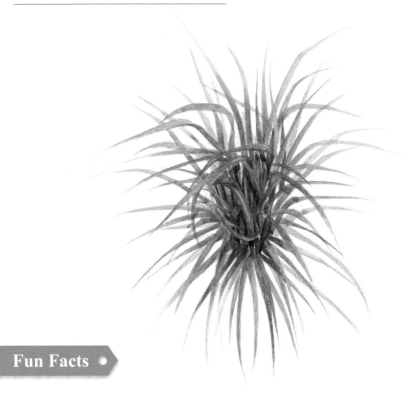

How is Ning Meng Cao (lemongrass) essential oil extracted?

The most common method for extracting Ning Meng Cao essential oil is steam distillation. The specific procedure involves placing flowers, leaves, peels and roots of Ning Meng Cao in a distillation apparatus. Steam is then introduced, causing the aromatic oil and water to distill simultaneously. After cooling through a condenser, the water is separated, leaving behind the extracted oil known as Ning Meng Cao essential oil.

Chinese Common Names: Xiang Mao, Xiang Ma, Ning Meng Mao

Latin Name: *Cymbopogon citratus* Stapf

The Legend of Ning Meng Cao

Legend has it that there was a beautiful angel in heaven named Xue Ning, and she especially loved the earthly realm, yearning to experience human life.

One day, Xue Ning finally descended to the earthly realm and landed in a field of lemongrass. She felt overjoyed and danced gracefully amid the sweet fragrance of Ning Meng Cao. At that moment, a handsome prince happened to pass by on his white horse. The prince with his sapphire-like eyes instantly caught sight of Xue Ning. He was stunned by her beauty and fell in love with her at first sight.

Collecting himself, the prince approached and greeted her. With a glance, Xue Ning also fell in love with him. Afterward, the two spent a period of affectionate and enviable days on the earthly realm.

However, their bliss was short-lived. Their relationship was known by the heavenly deity who governed the divine realms, and he was furious. There had always been a rule: humans and angels were not allowed to fall in love. If they did, their affection would be severed, and they would be forever encased in the Ice Forest of Shadows.

Refusing to let go of their love, the prince and Xue Ning pleaded with the heavenly deity to allow them to remain together. Touched by their love, the deity transformed their hearts and affection into Ning Meng Cao. The language of Ning Meng Cao's flower is the unspoken love.

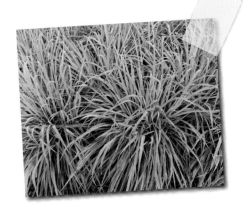

The heavenly deity also bestowed a blessing upon the Ning Meng Cao: if two lovers possessed it, they could be together forever.

Gua Lou

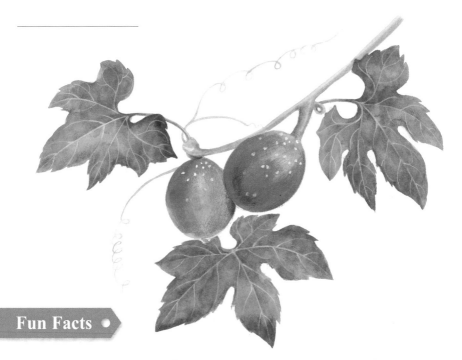

Is Tian Hua Fen powdery?

Speaking of "Tian Hua Fen", some people may think it is a powdery substance. Tian Hua Fen is a traditional Chinese medicine which refers to the chunky roots of the plant Gua Lou in the Cucurbitaceae family. Despite its name containing the word "powder" in Chinese, it is not actually in a powdery form.

In the Ming Dynasty (1368-1644 AD), Chen Jiamo (a famous doctor in ancient China) believed that the root of Gua Lou was named Tian Hua Fen because the stripes inside its root were naturally formed. Li Shizhen, on the other hand, thought that the root of Gua Lou was as white as snow when it was ground into fine powder. Hence, he referred to the root of Gua Lou as Tian Hua Fen.

Chinese Common Names: Gua Lou, Yao Gua

Latin Name: *Trichosanthes kirilowii* Maxim.

The Story of Gua Lou

During the Qing Dynasty (1616-1911 AD), in the mountains of northern China, there was a village where a 15-year-old boy lived with his poor mother. Life was difficult for them.

One night, the boy had a dream in which an old man with a white beard told him, "We are neighbors, I live right across from your house. Come and visit me when you have time!"

The next morning, the boy went to the designated spot but found nothing. As he stood there in confusion, he noticed small green shoots emerging from the wild grass. He carefully cleared the surrounding weeds and checked on them regularly, fearing they might be eaten by livestock. The vines grew vigorously, eventually bearing some small green melons. He treated it like a treasure, being too cautious to touch them.

As autumn arrived, the round melons turned orange, resembling pumpkins. One night, he dreamed of the white-bearded old man again. With a smile, the old man said, "Young man, you are a diligent and kind person. You've treated me well. Tomorrow you can pick those melons and sell them to Tongjitang Pharmacy!" Following the advice of the old man, the boy indeed made a considerable amount of money. The pharmacy explained that these melons were called Gua Lou whose roots and seeds were used for medicinal purposes.

The boy and his mother planted more Gua Lou in their courtyard, and within a few years, they became rich. They also generously taught other poor people how to cultivate it and helped the entire community to improve their livelihoods.

Tian Men Dong

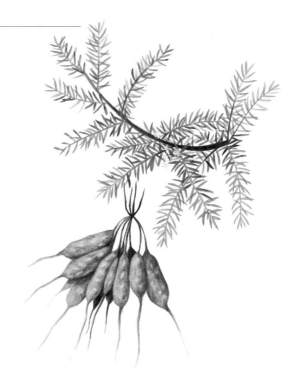

How to grow Tian Men Dong?

1. Buy Tian Men Dong's seeds, sow them in the pot in February or March, and keep them indoors at room temperatures of 14°C to 18°C. This plant thrives in moist, fertile and loose soil. One month after sowing, the seeds will sprout.When their stems and vines become dense, they can be cut and placed separately into the new potted soil to produce new plants.

2. Plant fresh tuberous roots of Tian Men Dong directly. The whole part of the root grows quickly. Therefore, in addition to replenishing new potted soil, some of the old roots and aging stems need to be pruned as well in early spring each year.

Chinese Common Names: San Bai Bang, Si Dong, Lao Hu Wei Ba Gen

Latin Name: *Asparagus cochinchinensis* Merr.

The Story of Tian Men Dong

In the late Ming Dynasty (1368-1644 AD), there was a large-scale peasant uprising led by the leader named Li Zicheng. He wanted to team up with the great general Zhang Xianzhong to overthrow the corrupt Ming Dynasty. To do this, Li Zicheng decided to visit Zhang Xianzhong in person.

However, when Li Zicheng arrived for his visit, he was told that Zhang Xianzhong's wife was giving birth. Therefore, Zhang Xianzhong had to send his assistant to greet Li Zicheng instead.

Growing impatient and yet to meet Zhang Xianzhong after a considerable wait, Li Zicheng got so mad that he slammed his fist on the table and shouted, "How could Zhang Xianzhong still not meet me!"

The assistant got frightened. While telling the servants what to do, the assistant hurriedly said, "Please, General Li, don't be angry. General Zhang can't leave his wife alone right now. May I interest you in some delicacies? General Zhang will come to you shortly."

While listening to the assistant's apology, he was served with a plate of tea snacks, which were crystal clear and jade-like, with an inviting aroma. Curious, he asked, "What is this?"

The assistant replied, "This is called candied Tian Men Dong, please have a try."

While trying these snacks, Li Zicheng was pleasantly surprised to find that they were sweet, refreshing, and so soft that they melted in his mouth. As a result, Li Zicheng let go of his anger and exclaimed, "Wow, these are really tasty!"

Calming down, Li Zicheng was informed by the assistant, "Tian Men Dong is not only tasty but also good for your health. It nourishes Yin and moistens the lungs, and also clears lung heat. Please wait for another moment, General Zhang would come soon."

Shortly thereafter, Zhang Xianzhong, having just celebrated the birth of his child, arrived in the living room and was eager to discuss their strategy against the Ming Dynasty with Li Zicheng.

He Shou Wu

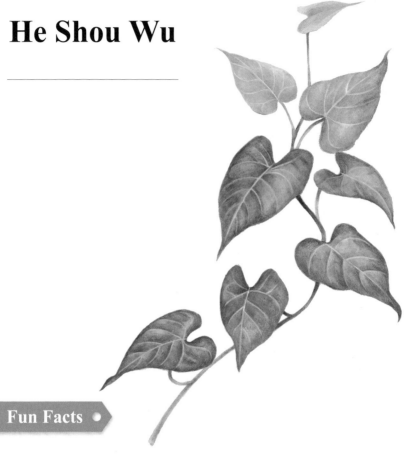

Why are the stalks and stems of He Shou Wu called Ye Jiao Teng (vines that tangle in the night)?

Legend has it that during the night, even if separated by over 1 meter, the stalks and stems of He Shou Wu would intertwine with each other. They would remain tangled for a considerable time before naturally separating. This process of tangling and separating repeats three or four times throughout the night. Hence, the stalks and stems of He Shou Wu are also known as Ye Jiao Teng, meaning vines that tangle in the night.

Chinese Common Names: Duo Hua Liao, Zi Wu Teng, Ye Jiao Teng

Latin Name: *Pleuropterus multiflorus* Nakai

　　　　　The Legend of He Shou Wu

A long time ago, some local officials were always bossing around poor villagers, forcing them to do hard labor.

Hidden away in an unknown mountain, there was a village, home to a poor peasant with weathered dark skin and snow-white hair. Unfortunately, one day he was press-ganged into doing the hard labor. From dawn till dusk, he had to toil away on the rugged slopes. When night fell, he was locked in a dark, dreary cell, often suffering from hunger pangs.

One night, as he was suffering from hunger, he noticed that there were many vines creeping into the cell. With a growling belly and nothing to eat, he plucked at the leaves to eat. From then on, every night, he relied on this unknown plant to keep from starving.

Fortune finally smiled upon him. He was set free from the harsh labor. He then gratefully uprooted this unknown plant, wrapped it up tight, and brought it home through thick and thin. Seeing his return, the villagers couldn't believe their eyes. Despite years of hardship, he looked younger than before. His hair became black again and his complexion got brightened. The villagers were very curious and asked him for his secrets. Revealing this mysterious plant wrapped in cloth, the farmer explained, "This plant saved me from starving every night when I was jailed." Since no one knew its name, they decided to call it "He Shou Wu" in honor of the peasant's surname "He".

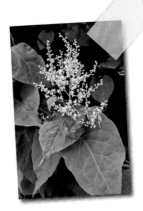

Fu Fang Teng

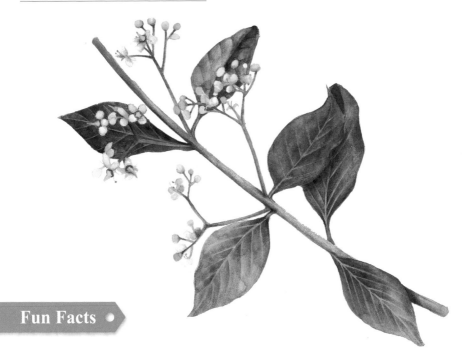

The multifaceted green sprite: Fu Fang Teng

Fu Fang Teng can cover the ground, twine around trees, and even climb walls. This climbing plant, capable of maximizing space utilization and improving green coverage, is an excellent choice for vertical gardening. Not only does it enjoy rapid growth and strong sprouting abilities, but it also boasts robust ecological functions. It is also highly resistant to pruning, easy to maintain and water-saving.

Furthermore, Fu Fang Teng is able to absorb harmful gases like sulfur dioxide, sulfur trioxide, chlorine, hydrogen fluoride, and nitrogen dioxide. This makes it an ideal plant for greening industrial areas facing severe air pollution.

Chinese Common Names: Huan Gu Jin, Pa Teng, Pa Xing Wei Mao

Latin Name: *Euonymus fortunei* Hand.-Mazz.

The Story of Fu Fang Teng

Once upon a time, in a humble farmhouse, there lived a poor family with four kids. They are so poor that relying solely on farming wasn't enough to support them all. As a result, the father decided to venture into mountains to find some precious herbs to provide for the family.

At first, it was easy for him to find valuable herbs like Ling Zhi. But soon, everyone in the village caught on, and herb-hunting became the latest hit. It became increasingly harder for him to find anything worthwhile.

One day, he went up the mountain to find herbs but returned empty-handed. As he saw his frail kids, he felt a pang of sadness. That night, he discussed with child's mother and made a decision to go deeper into the mountains in search of more valuable herbs.

Bright and early the next day, the father set out with some provisions. He managed to reach into the depths of the mountain after a few hours' journey. He spotted a large, precious herb growing on a steep cliff. Determined, he began to climb. But a slip left him with a hurt leg. Unable to walk, he reached for nearby plants, crushing and applying them to his leg. After a while, feeling better, he slowly made his way home.

Later, he dug this miraculous plant out and planted it at home. Every time he ventured into the mountains thereafter, he carried some of this plant with him in case of injuries. Soon, word spread about its healing properties, and it became known as Huan Gu Jin (bone-healing vine) in some places.

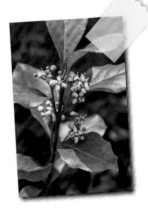

Shan Qian Niu

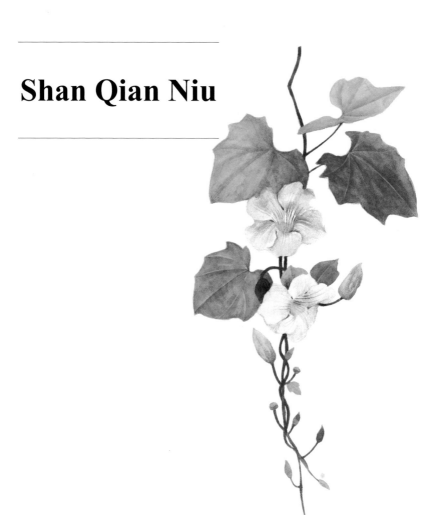

Do you know why Shan Qian Niu is also called Bengal Clockvine?

Shan Qian Niu, originated from Bangladesh, can reach to heights of above 7 meters and stretch over 20 meters. It has strong climbing capabilities. It is dubbed "Bengal Clockvine" due to the fact that it twines around a support in a clockwise direction.

Chinese Common Names: Da Hua Shan Qian Niu, Da Hua Lao Ya Zui, Bengal Clockvine

Latin Name: *Thunbergia grandiflora* Roxb.

The Story of Shan Qian Niu

Once upon a time, in a village, there lived a very cocky man who liked to venture into the mountains to catch snakes. Since he had never failed in his hunt, he proudly proclaimed himself the "best snake-catcher" of the village. He frequently boasted about his abilities and held a disdainful attitude toward other snake catchers.

There were times when the villagers were puzzled as their livestock, including chickens and sheep, began to disappear. However, it didn't take long before they realize a snake was the culprit. Despite their efforts, the cunning snake managed to escape away several times. Frustrated and out of options, the villagers turned to the self-proclaimed "best snake-catcher" for help. He strutted to the snake's den, setting up traps to lure it out. However, instead of being caught, the snake bit him, causing him to writhe in pain on the ground. Just then, another young man passing by witnessed this scene. Without hesitation, he grabbed some trumpet-shaped plants, crushed and applied them to the wound of the snake-catcher. Fortunately, the pain faded away.

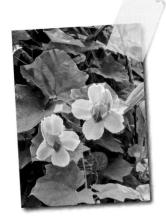

Later on, this young lad helped catch this snake. He also revealed that the plant he used could treat snake bites. Because it looked like morning glories and grew in the mountains, the villagers started to call it "Shan Qian Niu", meaning a plant resembles morning glory flowers growing in the mountains.

Bi Li

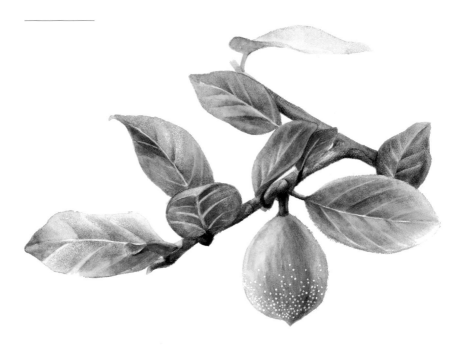

The Ingredient for White Grass Jelly: Bi Li

Hey kids, have you ever tried white grass jelly? White grass jelly are made from the seeds of Bi Li. First, you have to pick some Bi Li and take the seeds out. Then you can wrap them up in cloth and squeeze them in some cool water until you get the gel out of the seeds. After that, you can add a bit of coagulant, let it set and there it is! You have got yourself some crystal-clear white grass jellies. Especially on hot summer days, nothing beats a chilled bowl of these delicious treats!

Chinese Common Names: Liang Fen Zi, Mu Lian, Liang Fen Guo
Latin Name: *Ficus pumila* L.

The Story of Bi Li

Once upon a time, in the beautiful Taiwan, there lived a lovely girl named Ai Yu. Her village was very poor, and her parents could not afford to raise her. As a result, they had to send Ai Yu to work in a wealthy family.

One day, while Ai Yu was carrying some packages from the wealthy family to the village, her belly rumbled loudly as she was passing by a clear stream. Spotting an orange thing floating on the water, she causally scooped it up and found it soft and translucent. After careful observation, she decided to eat it to ease her hunger. To her surprise, it was incredibly sweet and tasty.

Curious about where this yummy food came from, she carefully observed the surroundings. Along the riverbank, she found a vine's fruits falling into the river and they turned into the same orange thing she just ate.

Ai Yu was excited. She took this orange thing to the village and shared her discovery with the villagers. Soon, everyone in the village caught on and went to try this tasty food. From then on, this special treat was named "Ai Yu".

As time went on, people learned that the vine's fruit is called Liang Fen Guo, the translucent thing that is edible is called Liang Fen (grass jelly), and the plant producing this fruit is called Bi Li.

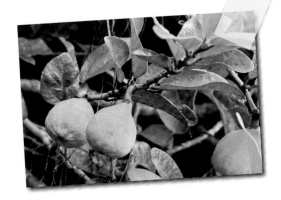

Ge

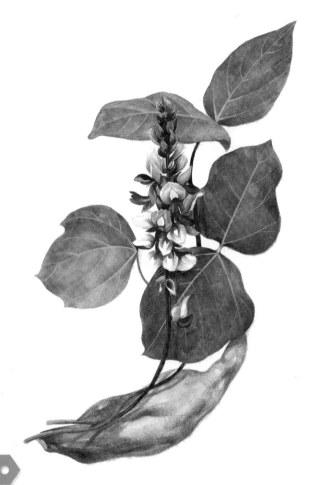

How to choose Ge Gen (the root-tuber of Ge)?

1. Check the color. The exterior of genuine Ge Gen is white or light brown skin, and sometimes covered with pieces of brown skin. Fake Ge Gen, on the other hand, has a brownish surface with irregular small cracks, longitudinal wrinkles, and inconspicuous pore-like protrusions.

2. Check the smell. Genuine Ge Gen has no distinct odor and tastes slightly sweet, while the fake one may have a slight odor but tastes somewhat bitter.

Chinese Common Names: Ye Ge (wild kudzu vine), Ge Teng (kudzu vine)
Latin Name: *Pueraria montana* var. *lobata*

The Story of Ge

Legend has it that during the flourishing period of the Tang Dynasty (618-907 AD), there lived a couple at the foot of a mountain. The husband, Fu Lang, devoted himself to studying for the imperial civil examination, while his wife, She Nv, worked diligently in the fields. After ten years of study, Fu Lang was finally awarded Jinshi (a successful candidate in the highest imperial civil examinations of ancient China). However, instead of being overjoyed, Fu Lang was not in the mood. Here is the thing. In the bustling city of Chang'an, Fu Lang had come across many fancy ladies from rich families. Every lady is as beautiful as blooming flowers with their lush figures and radiant beauty. When Fu Lang thought of his wife, who became frail and skinny due to years of hard work, he got a crazy idea of divorcing She Nv and marrying someone "better". Then he sent a letter home through a fellow villager, and it contained just two lines of poetry expressing his thoughts of divorcing. When She Nv figured out the connotation of the poetry, she was heartbroken. Her tears flowed like a never-ending river. Food became the last thing on her mind, and her once cheerful face turned all gloomy.

However, the mountain deity, touched by She Nv's story, guided her in a dream to dig Ge Gen and eat it every day, and it worked like magic. She Nv soon turned into a beautiful and glowing lady.

Meanwhile, Fu Lang realized his decision was so stupid and irresponsible. How could he abandon his wife, who had shared joys and sorrows with him for many years? As a result, he hurried back home to apologize to his wife, only to find his wife exceptionally beautiful. Overjoyed, the couple reunited and enjoyed their happy and prosperous life together. Since then, women of the She nationality, where She Nv came from, started a new tradition — eating Ge Gen. This tradition makes nearly every one of them voluptuous, slender, and fair-skinned.

Hua Nan Ren Dong

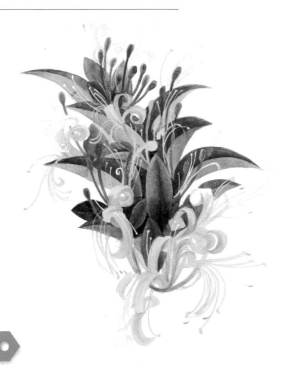

What other interesting names does Hua Nan Ren Dong have?

Hua Nan Ren Dong blooms in March, producing a subtle scent with red pedicels. Initially, the flowers bloom white and gradually turn yellow over the course of a day or two, hence earning itself the name "Jin Yin Hua", meaning a flower with both gold and silver colors. Additionally, it is a flower with one stalk bearing two blossoms, and the stamens of two blossoms pair together like a lovely couple, just as a pair of "Yuan Yang", or mandarin ducks (a symbol of eternal love in Chinese culture) flying and dancing together. As a result, it is also named "Yuan Yang Teng".

Chinese Common Names: Da Jin Yin Hua, Shan Jin Yin Hua, Tu Yin Hua

Latin Name: *Lonicera confusa* DC.

The Legend of Jin Yin Hua

Around fifteen hundred years ago, in what is now Henan Province, there existed a place called Huangchi, where a renowned physician named Dr. Huang lived. His twin daughters, Xiao Jinhua and Xiao Yinhua, were as beautiful as blooming flowers. The Huang family was respected by the villagers for their generosity and kindness.

One day, a dreadful plague swept through the village, spreading terror and despair. Despite Dr. Huang's tireless efforts, his antidotes proved powerless against the relentless disease. Witnessing the suffering of the villagers, the sisters made a courageous choice. Without their father's permission, they journeyed to the Temple of the Medicine God in Qinglong Town and made a heartfelt vow to find a cure for the plague, no matter the cost. Moved by their bravery, the Medicine God worked his enchantment, turning the sisters into a flower with one stalk bearing two blossoms. He then appeared in Dr. Huang's dream, guiding him to bring back the flower. Bright and early the next day, Dr. Huang went to the temple to gather the flower. Following the divine instruction, he brewed the flower into a pot of tea and then shared it with the villagers. And then, a magical thing happened, the miracle tea worked wonders, curing the diseases of all.

When the villagers learned that the life-saving tea came from the sacrifice of Xiao Jinhua and Xiao Yinhua, they flooded into the temple to express their gratitude. In honor of the courageous sisters, they named that miraculous flower after the sisters' names — Jin Yin Hua, also known as "Er Hua", or twin blooms.

According to legend, the Jade Emperor, the supreme ruler of Heaven, was deeply moved upon hearing their heroic deed. He crowned them as the Flower Fairies of Jin Yin Hua, forever guarding their beloved homeland with the Medicine God.

Shui Fei Ji

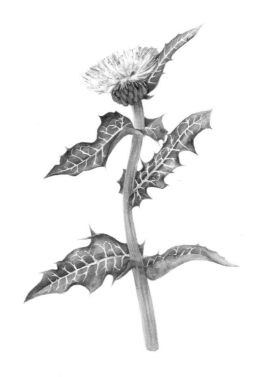

Let's have an experiment on the temperature of Shui Fei Ji seed germination

1. Put freshly harvested Shui Fei Ji seeds in petri dishes lined with four layers of gauze for germination experiments, with 30 seeds per group. Place the petri dishes in constant temperature incubators of 5-10°C, 16-25°C, and 28-34°C respectively. Observe the time and conditions of the germination of the seeds. The experiment should be repeated 3 times before calculating the average germination rate for each incubator.

2. The experiment reveals that the optimal germination temperature for Shui Fei Ji seeds is 16-25°C. Germination behavior is inhibited at temperatures below 10°C or above 30°C. During the germination and growth process, it is observed that seeds begin to sprout after 6 days in the incubator at 16-25°C with a germination rate of 94%.

Chinese Common Names: Shui Fei Zhi, Nai Ji, Lao Shu Jin
Latin Name: *Silybum marianum* Gaertn.

The Legend of Shui Fei Ji

In the early 1900s in Germany, there were many mushroom hunters who roamed the lush mountains in search of mushrooms. Hidden among the sturdy trees like beech, oak, and hazel, or tucked away in the secret hideouts of decaying wood and under the carpet of fallen leaves, a variety of mushrooms awaited discovery.

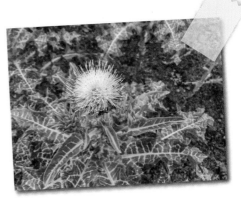

However, in these lush mountains, mushroom hunters may encounter with poisonous mushrooms. With caps of green or gray, these mushrooms masqueraded as harmless with a smooth edge, round shape, fibrous inner surface, a white stalk, and a prominent volva. However, they were the deceptive "Death Cap", a toxic mushroom similar to edible mushrooms and capable of causing liver failure and death. Many people died from eating this "Death Cap" accidentally.

Fortunately, a mushroom enthusiast who, in a stroke of luck, stumbled upon a magical herb with upright and ridged stems, branching as well as small purple flowers boasting delicate stamens. This herb, known as Shui Fei Ji, exudes a milk white bitter juice when its stem is cut open. Remarkably, those who consumed this herb before consuming poisonous mushrooms were shielded from the venomous effects of the deadly mushrooms. News of this miraculous discovery spread like wildfire among the mushroom hunters, saving countless lives from then on.

Because the stems of this herb exude a milky white juice when it is cut open, it is also known as "Niu Nai Ji", or Milk Thistle.

Yi Mu Cao

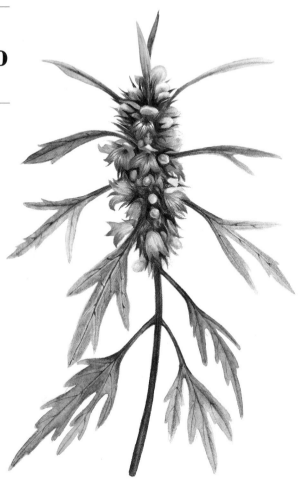

What does the shoot of Yi Mu Cao look like?

When in its infancy, Yi Mu Cao lacks stem and has basal, heart-shaped leaves with shallow serrated edges resembling gentle waves. Its long leaf stalks look like several small fans. With a verdant hue, Yi Mu Cao is also called "Tong Zi Cao".

Chinese Common Names: Yi Mu Hao (it means motherwort herb.), Yi Mu Hua (it means motherwort flower.), Ji Mu Cao

Latin Name: *Leonurus japonicus* Houttuyn

The Story of Yi Mu Cao

Once upon a time, there was a young man who, despite years of efforts, failed to achieve the highest honor in the imperial civil examination in ancient China after repeated attempts. Disheartened by his failures, he drowned his sorrows in alcohol all day long. Meanwhile, his mother, deeply worried about him, fell seriously ill, and remained bedridden for months despite numerous attempts by various doctors to cure her. The young man, who was desperate to save his mother, was at a loss.

One day, while walking on the street, he came across a fortune teller who spoke of a skilled physician living at the foot of the northern green hills, possibly being capable of curing his mother. The hills were far from his home, the journey was perilous, and the truthfulness of the fortune teller's words were uncertain. Though the villagers advised against it, fueled by his love for his mother, the young man was determined to find a cure and set out on the journey.

When arriving at the foot of the hills, he discovered the physician, whose yard was filled with all types of herbs. The physician, touched by the young man's filial piety, shared with him a collection of herbs and a handful of seeds. After expressing his gratitude, the young man hurried home, determined to save his mother. When he returned, he promptly brewed the herbs for his mother, and his mother recovered a lot within few days.

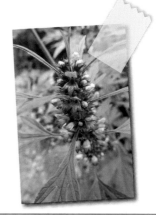

Villagers came to ask about the miracle medicine, and the young man shared the seeds with the villagers. Soon, women in the village found relief from gynecological issues. Since the herb was discovered by the young man to heal his mother and it would also benefit other women, people called it "Yi Mu Cao", or motherwort.

Wen Shu Lan

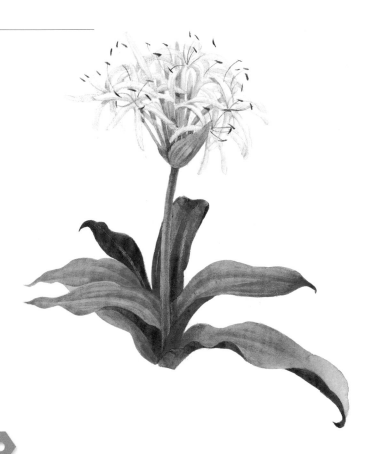

The Natural Bandage: Wen Shu Lan

In the depths of the mountains, if you get lost, injured, or have a bone fracture, you can pick the leaves of Wen Shu Lan and beat it with rocks to make it soften. After heating them with fire, you can get a natural bandage.

Chinese Common Names: Bai Hua Shi Suan, Luo Qun Dai, Wen Lan Shu
Latin Name: *Crinum asiaticum* var. *sinicum* Baker

The Legend of Wen Shu Lan

According to legend, back in the 6th century BC, Wen Shu Pu Sa (Manjushri Bodhisattva) emerged mischievously from his mother's right rib to come into this world. He was born with a golden purple glow, and he couuld speak without learning, just like a fairy boy. Adorned with the seven treasures, he brought blessings to the earthly realm. Revered as "Great Wisdom Wen Shu Pu Sa", he embodied wisdom and eloquence, being the epitome of intellect.

Of all the competitions in the world, the battle of intelligence is the ultimate one. Think of it like this ancient Greek saying, "Wisdom grows three leaves in its garden: good thoughts, good words, and good deeds". Wen Shu Lan represents keen insight and pure heart and therefore it is very suitable to compare Wen Shu Pu Sa with Wen Shu Lan. Wen Shu Lan has deep connections with Buddhism, gracing Buddhist temples with its dignified presence. Drenched in Wen Shu Pu Sa's magic, it radiates nobility, grace, and beauty, capturing hearts far and wide. So naturally, it's named "Wen Shu Lan".

As summer swelters and flowers play hide-and-seek, Wen Shu Lan steps up to the plate. Its long stems hoist up fluffy white blooms like elegant umbrellas, standing tall and proud. The stamens emit a pleasant scent, together with the scent of Buddhism temples, telling people to find inner peace.

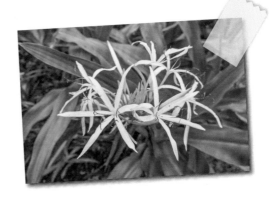

Da Che Qian

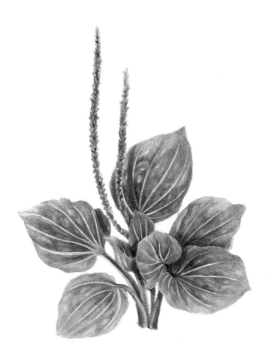

The Morphological Differences between Da Che Qian and Xiao Che Qian

Da Che Qian:

(1)A perennial herbaceous plant; (2)It has short and stout rhizomes with fibrous roots; (3)The leaves are upright, either ovate or broadly ovate in shape, with an acute tip, and they may have wavy margins or irregular serrations; (4)The flower stalk is erect, reaching heights of 15 to 120 centimeters; (5)The capsule is elliptical in shape; (6)The number of seeds ranges from 8 to 18, and they are brown or brownish in color.

Xiao Che Qian:

(1)An annual herbaceous plant; (2)Its roots are cylindrical in shape; (3)The leaves can be upright or spreading, with an elliptical, elliptical-lanceolate, or lanceolate-ovate shape; (4)The flowers are curved, with lengths ranging from 4 to 17 centimeters; (5)The capsule is conical in shape; (6)The seeds are black-brown.

Chinese Common Names: Qian Guan Cao, Da Ye Che Qian, Da Zhu Er Duo Cao
Latin Name: *Plantago major* L.

The Story of Che Qian Cao

During the Western Han Dynasty (206 BC-25 AD), there was a great general named Ma Wu. Once, while leading his army on a border expedition, they became trapped by enemy forces in a deserted land. The scorching sun beat down relentlessly, without a drop of rain falling from the sky. With supplies running low, many soldiers and their horses died from hunger and thirst. Those who survived suffered from severe abdominal swelling due to hunger and thirst, and their urine turned red like blood. When they urinated, they experienced excruciating pain and

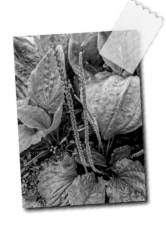

discomfort. Even the surviving horses struggled and whinnied in pain while urinating. The army physician diagnosed it as hematuria, a condition requiring medication to clear heat and promote urination. However, the physician was helpless due to the lack of such medicine.

Ma Wu had a horse groomer named Zhang Yong. Zhang Yong and the three horses under his care also suffered from hematuria, enduring immense pain.

One day, Zhang Yong noticed that his three horses were no longer urinating blood, and their spirits were greatly lifted. Curious, he watched closely and discovered they were nibbling on a wild grass that looked like big pig's ears. He then plucked some and boiled it into a potion. After a few days of drinking it, he felt better, and his urine returned to normal.

Excited by this discovery, Zhang Yong reported it to Ma Wu. Delighted, Ma Wu immediately ordered the entire army to consume the potions made by this plant that resembled big pig's ears, which was also called "Da Zhu Er Duo Cao".

Because this plant was found in front of the cart, people began to call it "Che Qian Cao", meaning a plant growing in front of the cart.

Ye Ju

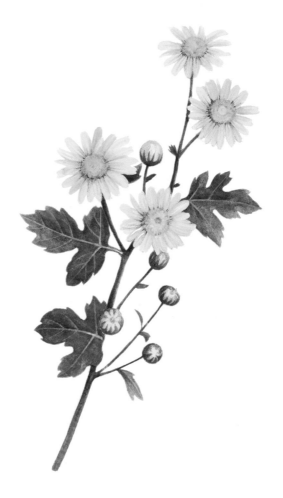

Do you know what is behind the beauty of Ye Ju?

Ye Ju possesses a simple beauty. It thrives in the mountains, with soft hues and a delicate fragrance. Ye Ju blooming in the autumn, it is often used to symbolize the noble character of not being contaminated by the world and unyielding firmness.

Chinese Common Names: Huang Ju Zai, Lu Bian Huang, Shan Ju Hua

Latin Name: *Chrysanthemum indicum* L.

The Story of Ye Ju

Once upon a time, a young lad named Ah Niu lived near the tranquil banks of the Lu River. His father bid farewell to the world when he was just seven, leaving his hardworking mother to support their life by doing weaving work. Ah Niu's mother, burdened with grief, often wept, until her tears eventually robbed her of her sight.

When he grew up, Ah Niu hustled each day, peddling veggies to fund treatments for his mother's eyes. However, his mother's eyes remained veiled in darkness despite the large amount of money spent on her remedies.

One night, Ah Niu dreamed of a beautiful lady. Touched by his filial heart, she instructed him to find a Ye Ju somewhere in the mountains. The blossom of that plant held the power to heal his mother's illness. Waking with resolve, Ah Niu embarked on a quest for the elusive flower.

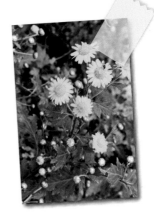

It was not until the afternoon that he finally found the plant, after he arrived at the place that the mysterious maiden had mentioned. There were nine flower buds on the stem, but only one flower had bloomed. As a result, Ah Niu uprooted it and carried this Ye Ju home. With tender care, he nurtured this plant, watering it diligently until all of the blossoms flourished. Each day, he plucked a bloom to brew a cup of tea for his mother. By the eighth day, his mother's eye illness recovered.

From this story, what we can learn is that Ye Ju has the remarkable ability to prevent eye diseases.

Ding Tou Guo

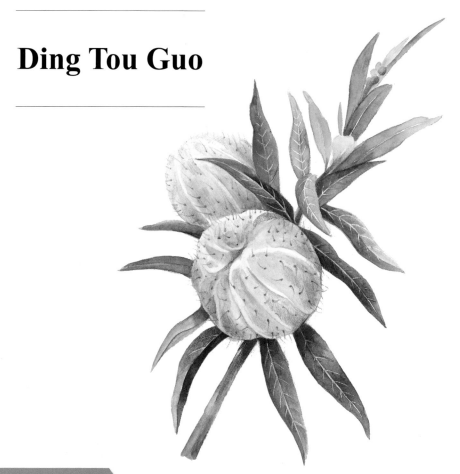

Fun Facts •

The Unusual Fruit: Ding Tou Guo

Ding Tou Guo is greenish-yellow in color with prickles on its surface. The fruit is very thin, with a hollow center, swollen into a spherical shape. When gently squeezed by hand, it is likely to release air, much like a small balloon. The fruit remains attached to the plant for a long time and can be used as an ornamental potted plant.

Chinese Common Names: Qi Qiu Hua, Qi Qiu Guo, Bang Tou Guo
Latin Name: *Gomphocarpus fruticosus* W. T. Ation

The Story of Ding Tou Guo

Once upon a time, there existed a beautiful island in the mystical Mediterranean Sea. Hot and dry in summer, warm and humid in winter, it flourished with lush green bushes and abundant subtropical fruits.

On the island, there lived a Jewish family whose parents were often busy with their trading ventures at sea. Their 10-year-old brother cared for his 4-year-old sibling. They would often go to the woods in search of fruits. The little brother, who was curious about every fruit, would often pluck strange fruits along the way and eat them without a second thought.

However, his indiscriminate consumption of fruits resulted in stomach troubles. Back home, the younger brother who looked pale from his upset stomach scared his older sibling.

Despite the discomfort, his tummy rumbled loudly because the diarrhea had emptied his stomach. Looking at the table, he noticed fruits with soft prickles on the peculiar branch. Once again, he stuffed them into his mouth without hesitation.

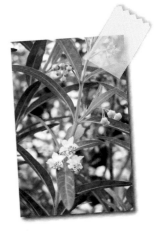

Shocked, the elder brother failed to stop his younger sibling from eating recklessly. Yet, to their surprise, the younger brother's diarrhea ceased after eating the fruit, and his rosy complexion began to return. This plant, bearing strange fruits with soft prickles like nails, was therefore called "Ding Tou Guo", meaning a fruit with nails on the surface.

Qing Xiang

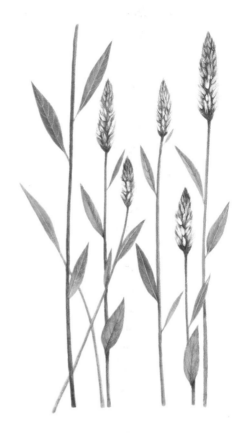

Do you know what Qing Xiang Zi (Qing Xiang's seed) looks like? Let's explore it together!

Qing Xiang Zi is the seed of Qing Xiang. Qing Xiang is harvested during the period from August to October. The above-ground parts or flower spikes are collected, sun-dried before we gently rub the flower spikes and remove impurities. Then, we can get Qing Xiang Zi as long as we sun-dried what we get from the flower spikes.

The dried Qing Xiang Zi is flattened and round, slightly thicker in the center than at the edges, with a diameter of 1-1.5 millimeters and a thickness of about 0.5 millimeters. The surface is smooth, black, and glossy. The seeds have thin and delicate skins, and thus easy to break. It has a white interior with a subtle odor.

Chinese Common Names: Ye Ji Guan Hua, Ji Guan Hua, Bai Ri Hong
Latin Name: *Celosia argentea* L.

The Story of Qing Xiang Zi

Legend has it that there was a hunter who ventured into the forest every day for his hunt. One day, amid the rustling leaves and chirping birds, he heard the faint cries echoing from the woods. Intrigued, he followed the sound until he stumbled upon a curious sight — a large, green box nestled among the grass. Approaching with caution, the hunter lifted the lid and made a surprising discovery — a young girl, whose clothes were worn and tattered, curled up inside the box.

Feeling sympathy for the poor girl, he rescued her from the box and took her home. He then asked why she would appear in the box. She revealed how her mother had fallen ill with a grave eye affliction and how she had sought help from two wandering healers who had promised a cure as long as the girl could guide them to find certain herbs in the mountain. Yet, their intentions were sinister, and they trapped her within the box, intending to abduct her.
Luckily, she was saved by the hunter.

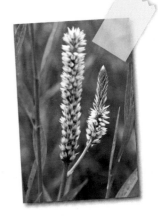

The hunter escorted the girl back home and promptly brewed a potion with the seeds of Ye Ji Guan Hua to help cure her mother. Some of it was ingested, while the rest was used to wash the eyes. Before long, the girl's mother's eyes recovered.

The villagers, after learning this story, began to call it "Qing Xiang" which meant the green box with Qing translated to green and Xiang to box. And the seed of Qing Xiang was known as "Qing Xiang Zi".

Shu Kui

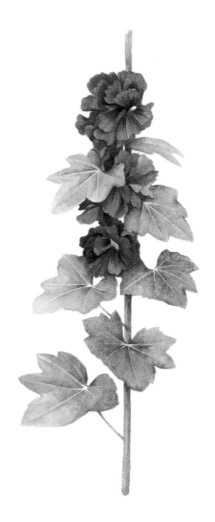

Why is Shu Kui also called Yi Zhang Hong?

Shu Kui is the city flower of Shuozhou City, Shaanxi Province. Its flowers are large, and the flowering phase is rather long. The locals call it "Da Hua". Shu Kui is also known as "Yi Zhang Hong", referring to its towering height of up to over 3 meters and its predominantly red blooms.

Chinese Common Names: Yi Zhang Hong, Ma Gan Hua, Dou Peng Hua
Latin Name: *Alcea rosea* L.

The Legend of Shu Kui

Once upon a time, there was a wealthy landowner who treated his servants with kindness. He married a pretty but delicate lady named Shu Kui. She was gentle and virtuous, and the man adored her very much.

Sadly, Shu Kui had always been in poor health. Despite the landowner's devoted care, her condition only worsened over time until, tragically, she passed away two years later.

This poor man was overwhelmed by grief and secluded himself in his room, refusing to eat or drink. His grief caused him to waste away, much to the concern of his servants. One night, Shu Kui appeared in his dream, promising to transform into flowers that would never leave his side.

When he woke up, he hurried to the courtyard and witnessed a miraculous scene: a plant with straight, towering stems and heart-shaped leaves. The thin stems were densely covered with exquisitely beautiful flowers, as lovely as his wife. Despite their ephemeral nature, these flowers bloomed tirelessly, unfurling their petals freely. As the gentle breeze caressed them, they seemed to nod and smile, just like his beloved wife.

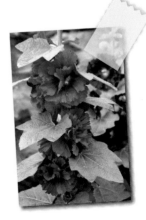

From then on, the landowner cared for the flowers as tenderly as he had cared for his wife. By the second year, the courtyard was overflowing with these blossoms, filling the air with their sweet fragrance. In memory of his wife, the landowner named the flowers after her — Shu Kui.

Wu Yue Ai

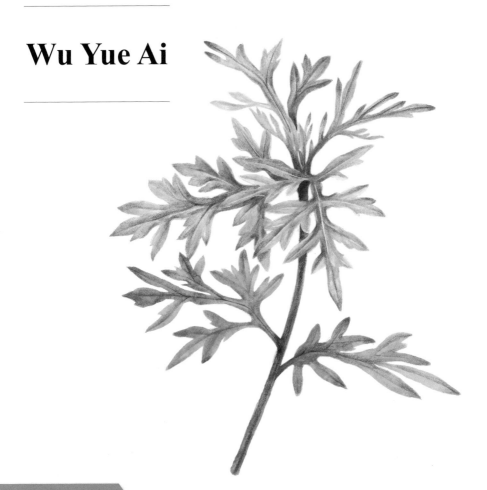

Why do we put Wu Yue Ai on the door on Dragon Boat Festival?

It is believed that Wu Yue Ai will bring good fortune and cure diseases. So people put it on the door for the health of the whole family.

Its leaves have been leveraged to treat disease, make food, and ward off evil and bad luck as a talisman from ancient times.

Chinese Common Names: Ai, Ye Ai Hao, Ai Ye
Latin Name: *Artemisia indica* Willd.

The Tale of Wu Yue Ai

In a prosperous year, one god who decided to investigate people's living condition dressed as a poor old man to look for some food. However, he was thrown out by a lady when begging her for leftovers.

The god was extremely mad. So he put a curse on the village that every villager would die of the plague. The lady realized that she had made a huge mistake, and the other villagers turned to blame her for what she had done.

The next morning, right before he spread the plague, the god saw a woman wading across the river with an older child in her arm and a younger one following her.

He felt very strange, so he decided to ask about it. The woman sighed and explained that she was taking these two children away from the plague. The older child was her stepchild, so she had to take good care of the children.

The god admired her very much, so he picked a few Wu Yue Ai and asked the woman to put them on windows or doors.

Then he conjured up a bridge to let them pass. The woman soon realized that the man in front of her was a god, so she thanked him, picked another bunch of the herb, and ran across the river through the magic bridge. Upon returning to the village, they put the herb on every door and window in the village.

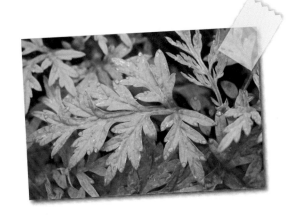

In the end, the villagers were all saved by this woman who was later appreciated by all.

Jie Geng

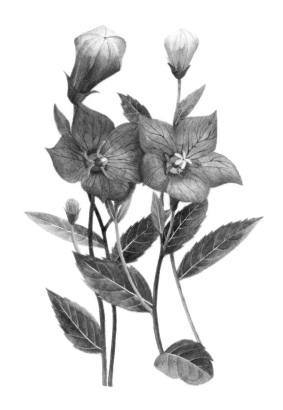

How does Jie Geng survive the winter?

Jie Geng's flower is called "Seng Guan Mao (monk hat)" or "Liu Jiao He (lotus in a hexagonal shape lotus)" since the flower is similar to a monk hat or lotus. It is a deep-rooting plant, so its root will grow thicker and thicker as time passes, and it can overwinter underground. After winter, new root will sprout from the old one. Besides, its seedlings can stand the winter at a temperature of −17°C.

Can it bloom twice a year?

Yes, of course! But you should prune it before the end of July after the first flowering, then strengthen the management of fertilizer and water to prevent and control pests and diseases timely, so that it can bloom again during early October.

Chinese Common Names: Ling Dang Hua, Bao Fu Hua, Seng Mao Hua
Latin Name: *Platycodon grandiflorus* A. DC.

The Tale of Jie Geng

A long time ago, a girl named Jie Geng who lost her parents lived in a village alone.

A boy who always played with Jie Geng told her that he would marry her once they grew up. Jie Geng agreed. The vow was made.

A few years later, they became a sweet couple. Then the boy had to go fishing in a remote place on a huge ship.

However, he never came back. She stood by the seaside waiting for him every single day, but the sea only brought sadness to her.

Decades later, Jie Geng became an old lady and her love still didn't turn up.

She cried, "God, please bring him back to me!"

Suddenly, a god appeared and spoke to her, "You are brokenhearted, so you must quit missing him."

"My heart will never change!" said the old lady.

"I already told you to stop missing him," sighed the god, "now I will condemn you to miss your love for eternity!"

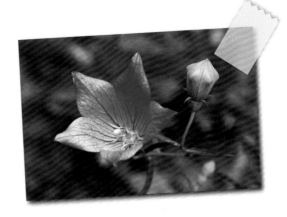

So she closed her eyes and turned into a beautiful flower.

Then people started to call this flower "Jie Geng", and it has been waiting for that boy by the seaside since then.

Chang Chun Hua

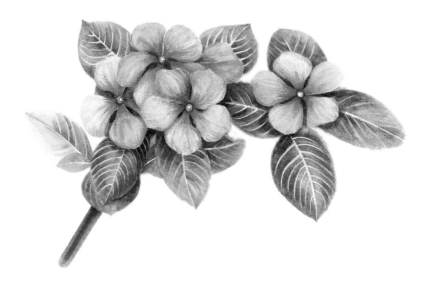

Chang Chun Hua is poisonous

Once a new leaf grows at the top of the tender branches, two flowers will emerge between the axils of the leaves, so Chang Chun Hua has many flowers. And since it blooms from spring to autumn without a break, it is also called "Ri Ri Chun (a flower with long flowering phase)". The vinblastine and vincristine in this flower can be extracted as chemotherapy medicines for various cancers, such as leukemia and Hodgkin's disease. But its whole plant is toxic, and it will reduce the leukocyte and thrombocyte in human blood, and cause muscle weakness, quadriplegia, and other symptoms after ingestion.

Chinese Common Names: Yan Lai Hong, Ri Ri Xin, Ri Ri Chun
Latin Name: *Catharanthus roseus* G. Don

The Tale of the Meizhanpo

There is a place called "Meizhanpo" in Jiujiang City, Jiangxi Province, and the name of the place is related to Chang Chun Hua.

During the Chongde period of the Qing Dynasty (1636-1643 AD), a businessman surnamed Mei, who had been doing business for many years, returned to Jiujiang City to settle down and opened a cloth store on the street near Meizhanpo. He was generous and treated people sincerely, so everyone wanted to buy clothes from him.

In addition to taking care of his business, Mr. Mei loved flowers and plants as well. In order to commemorate his first love, he planted dozens of Chang Chun Hua [people called it "Si Ji Mei (four-season flower)"] around his own house, and he even planted several rows of it in front of his store. This plant is known for its rapid growth, and it can cover the entire yard. Besides, one plant can have hundreds of flowers with extremely long flowering phases, showcasing its prosperity and vitality. In autumn, its flowers were still so dazzling when other flowers had withered. Those flowers could even survive the winter. The nearby residents loved this kind of plant so much that they came to collect seeds from Mr. Mei. And Mr. Mei was so kind-hearted and gave the seeds to them generously.

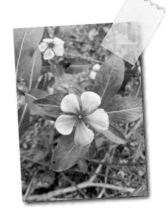

Moreover, those businessmen who are struggling with poor business believed that Chang Chun Hua must have brought good luck to Mr. Mei's business, so they planted this flower in front of their own stores as well. As a result, nearby streets were filled with Chang Chun Hua. And that is why this place is called "Meizhanpo".

San Qi

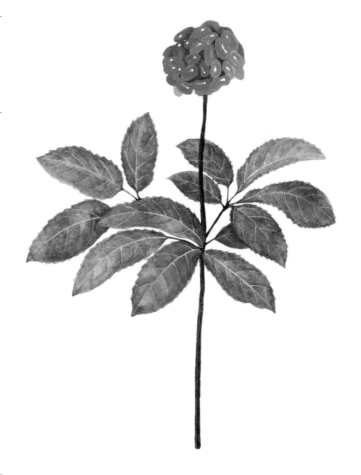

Do you know about San Qi?

San Qi is also known as Tian Qi, and its remarkable effects of dispersing blood stasis, stopping bleeding, and relieving swelling and pain have established itself as "Nan Guo Shen Cao (magical herb from the south)" and "Jin Bu Huan (more precious than gold)" since ancient times. Since it is often picked in spring and winter, it is also called "Chun (spring) Qi" or "Dong (winter) Qi".

Chinese Common Names: Tian Qi, Jin Bu Huan, Xue Jian Chou
Latin Name: *Panax notoginseng* F. H. Chen ex C. H. Chow

The Tale of San Qi

Once upon a time, a fairy named San Qi came to the human world to teach humans to grow plants.

One day, she was working in the farmland when a fierce black bear charging towards her. And a Miao (a Chinese ethnic group) young man named Ka Xiang killed the bear with an arrow and saved the fairy.

Ka Xiang came from an impoverished family and his mother had been ill for years. To thank Ka Xiang for saving her life, the fairy told him to look for a specific herb with leaves looking like her dress and branches like her belt, which could cure his mother's disease. His mother took this herb that Ka Xiang found for several times and really got cured.

Then he cured so many people with this herb.

People were utterly grateful. They asked the fairy, "What is this herb and why is it so magical?"

The fairy pointed at this herb and beamed, "How many branches and leaves does it have?"

People found that there were three branches and seven leaves.

"San Qi (numbers three and seven in Chinese)," one clever girl cried. So the name San Qi has been passed down for centuries to now.

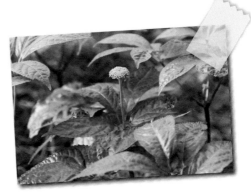

Da Ye Xian Mao

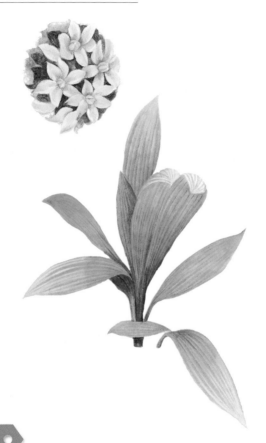

Let's observe Da Ye Xian Mao together

We can plant Da Ye Xian Mao's rhizome in a pot and observe when it blooms? And what color are its flowers?

Chinese Common Names: Du Mao Gen, Ye Zong, Jia Bin Lang Shu (fake *Areca catechu* L).

Latin Name: *Curculigo capitulata* O. Kuntze

The Origin of Da Ye Xian Mao

Li Shimin, one of emperors of the Tang Dynasty (618-907 AD), took many elixirs in order to maintain his youth, but none of them worked.

Li Shimin was not satisfied. Therefore, he announced that whoever found elixirs would be highly rewarded. The announcement soon spread throughout the whole country and to the Western Regions. One day, a Brahmin monk from a western country came and gave the emperor a tribute, which was shaped like garlic. After taking the elixir, Li Shimin felt extremely energetic and alive, and he even felt like he had become younger. The ministers were astonished as well and wondered what kind of magical medicine it was.

The monk revealed that its leaf looked like a Mao (thatch), and it grew in concealed places just like a fairy, so it was Xian Mao (fairy thatch).

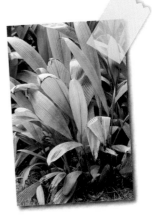

Li Shimin held a banquet for the monk as a reward, and then he hid the herb in the palace, which became an exclusive medicine for the emperor.

During the Kaiyuan period (713-741 AD) of the Tang Dynasty, the monk Tang Seng got to know this herb, and it was soon introduced to the rest of the country.

Ku Shen

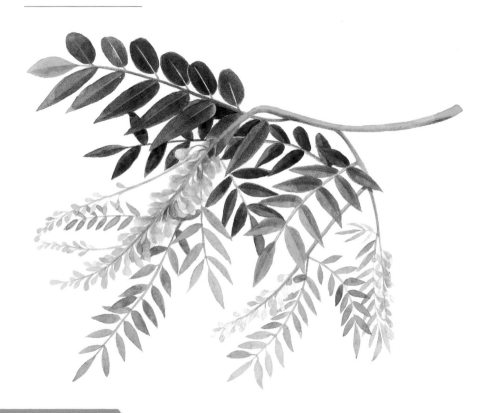

The Origin of Ku Shen's Name

How do you think the name "Ku Shen" comes into being? Does it taste bitter? Let me tell you a secret that it is called Ku Shen (bitter ginseng) since it tastes bitter and has a shape that is similar to ginseng.

Chinese Common Names: Di Huai, Bai Jing Di Gu, Shan Huai
Latin Name: *Sophora flavescens* Ait.

The Tale of Ku Shen

Once upon a time, there was a young cowboy whose parents had died herded cattle of the landlord for a living. He was covered with sores from his frequent walking on the wetlands.

Soon, the sores appeared on the landlord's family members. They believed that the disease came from the cowboy undoubtedly, so the landlord made an order to kill him.

Then the cowboy hid himself in a crack of a giant rock and never came out. Unfortunately, he was already dead when the villagers found him. They left him in the rock and sealed it with mud and stone hoping it would help him rest in peace.

However, another sores breakout and hit the village, none of the medicines could stop the unbearable itching. One night, the young cowboy told the villagers in a dream that there were many root-like herbs in the landslide area where he was buried, and those herbs could be boiled in water to drink or bathe so as to cure those sores. The villagers followed his instructions and the sores were eventually cured in days.

Upon hearing the news, the landlord decided to pick some herbs as well. He spotted some fruits that looked like rat droppings on the rock bushes. Then he took them home and boiled them in water. However, after drinking the herb water, the landlord died.

It is later discovered that the root-like herb picked by the villagers was Ku Shen's root, while the landlord took was Ku Shen Zi [*Brucea javanica* (L.) Merr.], which was poisonous.

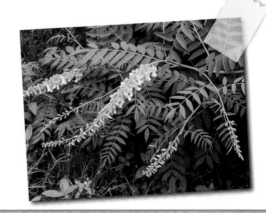

177

Long Ya Cao

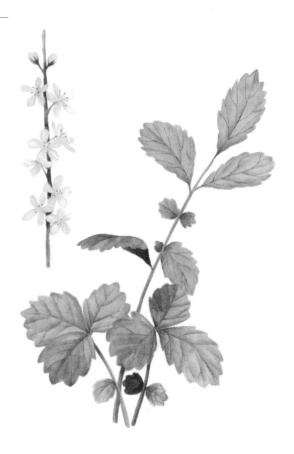

Xian He Cao can stop bleeding

Long Ya Cao is also known as Xian He Cao (heaven-sent crane herb). It can be used to stop bleeding. So if you accidentally cut yourself or start to bleed from a fall, you can rub it and apply it to the wound, which will soon stop the bleeding.

178

Chinese Common Names: Xian He Cao, Tuo Li Cao, Lao He Zui
Latin Name: *Agrimonia pilosa* Ledeb.

The Hemostatic Medicine: Xian He Cao

A long time ago, two Juren (ancient Chinese scholar who passed the imperial civil examination at the provincial level) were traveling to the capital to take further exams. Then the weather became extremely sweltering when they passed the beach area. The sun was blazing in the sky, making them sweaty, thirsty and exhausted.

All of a sudden, one of them had a nosebleed, which led to a rather panic moment since doctors and medicines were nowhere to be found in that deserted place. Seconds later, a heaven-sent crane with some herbs in its beak flew slowly over those two terrified people and dropped several herbs. The Juren who had a nosebleed picked those herbs up and started to chew them. Then his throat and mouth became moist and the nosebleed was cured. So they went on their way full of joy.

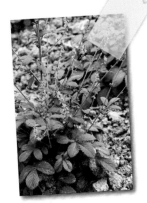

Later, both of them were awarded Jinshi (the successful candidate in the highest imperial civil examinations of ancient China) and became county officials of the seventh rank. However, they never forgot that magical experience. Therefore, they sent some people to look for those magical herbs in the mountains. In the end, those herbs were found, and it was confirmed that they could stop bleeding.

To commemorate the crane, people gave the herb the name "Xian He Cao (heaven-sent crane herb)", which was soon introduced to the public, listed in medicinal books, and widely used in disease treatment.

Hu Lu Cha

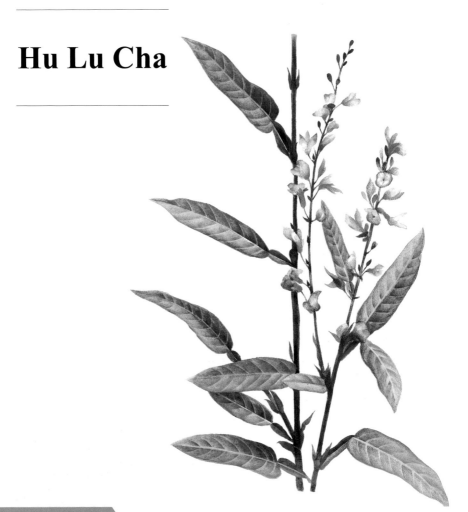

How to identify Hu Lu Cha?

What do you think Hu Lu Cha's leaf looks like? We can see that its leaf has two parts, one part is big and the other part is small. It looks just like a Hu Lu (gourd). So you will recognize it once you see its leaves, won't you?

Chinese Common Names: Bai Lao She, Niu Chong Cao, Lan Gou She
Latin Name: *Tadehagi triquetrum* Ohashi

Tales of the Herb ◦   **The Tale of Hu Lu Cha**

Once upon a time, there was a fish porter who delivered a package to one buyer after traveling dozens of miles.

On the way back, the weather became extremely sweltering. After arriving at a hill, he spotted a farmhouse, and an old lady was making hemp ropes under a tree nearby.

He asked the old lady for some water, the old lady gave him a bowl of herbal tea and said, "Young man, is this bowl enough for you?"

After thanking the old lady, he chugged the tea, and he felt energetic again very soon. He decided to pay for the tea with one copper coin, but he was rejected.

"We don't charge people for that tea since we drink it every day, and we always give it to passersby for free," said the old lady.

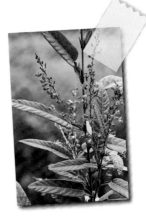

He expressed his heartful thanks to the old lady again. Then he asked her for the ingredients of the herbal tea and learned that it was made with the herb Hu Lu Cha growing near her house, whose leaves looked just like a gourd.

The porter went back home and told other people about that herb, and soon the herbal tea became popular.

Guangxi Di Bu Rong

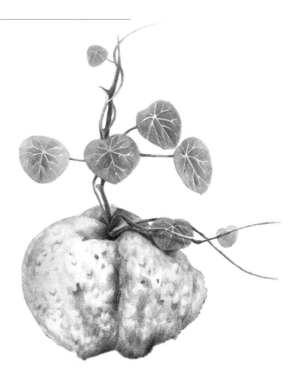

The Origin of the name of Guangxi Di Bu Rong

The huge lump on the ground is Guangxi Di Bu Rong's root. As a perennial deciduous vine plant, it has a succulent tuberous root, and the root tends to grow larger and larger until it breaks out of the ground, so it is called Di Bu Rong (out of the ground). It is also a beloved potted plant. Besides, it can be planted in soil or water. It is very easy to plant it in water, and what you need to do is to place its root hair in water.

Chinese Common Names: Shan Wu Gui, Jin Bu Huan, Di Dan

Latin Name: *Stephania kwangsiensis* H. S. Lo

The Tale of Shan Wu Gui

A long time ago, there was a small country called Yewang in southern China.

One summer, the army of Yewang lost the war against a powerful country. So the soldiers fled to a remote mountain with wounds and bruises, which was utterly unbearable. Due to the sweltering weather, many soldiers got eczema, and after experiencing a series of stomachaches and diarrhea, they finally collapsed.

All of a sudden, one soldier brought back a huge, round and tortoise-like herb, saying that it could be poisonous but there were no other choices. In the spirit of combating poison with poison, this soldier ate the herb doubtfully. Surprisingly, the herb worked and all of the discomforts were gone.

Then, the general ordered the soldiers to grind this herb into powders and put some into the food. Several days later, many soldiers didn't suffer from diarrhea or feel itchy and swelling and pain were gone.

They believed that God was helping them, so they felt refreshed and energetic all at once. At the general's order, the soldiers rushed out of the mountains like tigers, recaptured the lost territory and saved their own country.

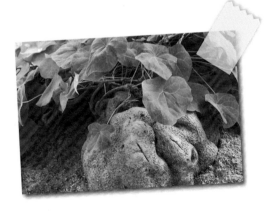

Since this herb had a huge root growing out of the ground, which looked just like a tortoise, the soldiers called it "Shan Wu Gui (tortoise in the mountain)" to commemorate it.

Luo Di Sheng Gen

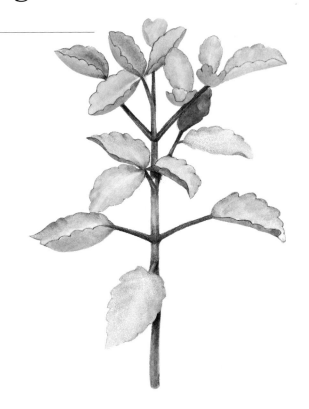

The Origin of Luo Di Sheng Gen

Do you know why it is called "Luo Di Sheng Gen (to take root upon landing)"? It boasts strong vitality, so it will take root upon landing on the ground. Let's give it a try! Now, put one of its leaves into the pot and wait for a few days. You will see that this leaf starts to take root with many small roots growing from the edge of it. What is even more surprising is that the new buds will sprout from those small roots, which will soon grow into a whole Luo Di Sheng Gen.

Chinese Common Names: Da Bu Si Cao, Ye Sheng Gen, Shai Bu Si
Latin Name: *Bryophyllum pinnatum* Oken

Strong Vitality — Da Bu Si Cao

Once upon a time, there was a young couple who loved each other deeply. A tribal leader had his eyes on the girl and tried to win her love with lavish gifts. However, the girl gave him a firm refusal, which infuriated the leader, so he took her home against her will. Invaluable gifts and money still didn't interest her. The girl choosed death as a testament to her unwavering resolve.

Her boyfriend was grief-stricken, so he swore on the grass at her grave, promising that he would seek justice for her. Before long, he delivered his promise and returned to her grave. Suddenly, the girl walked out of her grave that was covered by those grasses. Finally, the couple reunited.

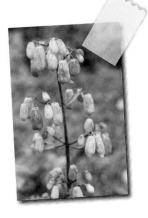

Later, they left their hometown, and only a few people saw them in remote places. It is said that they had been traveling around to provide medical care to people, and they were particularly good at treating bone pain and injuries, and even broken bones can be repaired perfectly. The magical medicine was the Da Bu Si Cao from the grave of the girl.

Su Tie

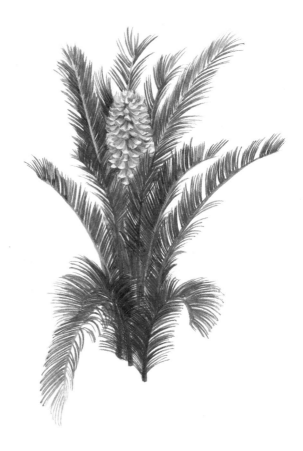

How to distinguish male Su Tie from female Su Tie?

Su Tie's trunk is as hard as iron, and it prefers fertilizers containing iron, so it is called Tie Shu (iron tree). Besides, the female and male flowers of Su Tie grow on separate plants, but it is easy to distinguish them. Its flower blooms at the top of the stem, the male flower looks like a large corn cob and the female one looks like a huge cabbage.

Su Tie is not only an ornamental plant, but can also be food or medicine. Its stem contains starch that is edible, and its seeds contain oil and abundant starch with slight toxicity, which can be made into food or medicine.

Chinese Common Names: Tie Shu, Pi Huo Jiao, Feng Wei Cao, Feng Wei Jiao
Latin Name: *Cycas revoluta* Thunb.

Tales of the Herb ●

The Origin of Tie Shu

A long time ago, there was a golden phoenix living in southern China, which boasted stunning feathers and a perfect singing voice.

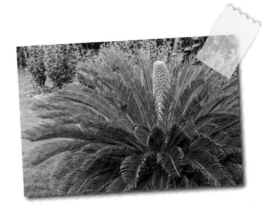

It would sometimes stand in the treetops or hover in the sky, singing beautiful songs to the hard-working people, showing them elegant dancing performances, so it was deeply loved by the people.

After hearing about the story of the phoenix, one government officer sent people to capture it, kept it in a cage, fed it with the most expensive and delicious food, and ingratiated it with every possible way so as to let it perform, but the phoenix remained silent.

After endless waiting, the officer became so mad that he burned the phoenix to death.

However, a small tree grew from the remaining ashes with hard bottle-green leaves that looked like the tail of the phoenix.

The phoenix was then admired by the people since they believed that the small tree was its reincarnation, so they called the plant "Tie Shu (iron tree)". Moreover, it was also called Feng Wei Jiao since it looked exactly like the phoenix's tail.

Tie Pi Shi Hu

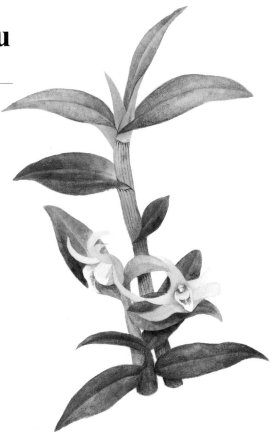

What are the benefits of consuming Tie Pi Shi Hu?

1. Tie Pi Shi Hu will nourish yin to keep fit and prolong life.

2. Tie Pi Shi Hu is helpful for women's beauty and skin-nourishing.

3. Tie Pi Shi Hu is suitable for improving sub-health state caused by excessive stress, overwork, and staying up late to work.

4. Tie Pi Shi Hu will help against constipation, acne, and dry mouth and tongue caused by poor circulation of body fluid.

Chinese Common Names: Lao Feng Dou, Tie Pi Lan, Yan Zhu
Latin Name: *Dendrobium catenatum* Lindl.

The Story of Tie Pi Shi Hu

Once upon a time, an emperor kept searching for an elixir for immortality every day. One day, a little Taoist accompanied by the emperor said he had a dream that an immortal descended to the mortal realm and spoke to him. Out of curiosity, the emperor asked the Taoist the details of the dream. The little Taoist replied that in his dream he found himself in a place with a broad ocean. And by the shore, there stood a mountain with many floating feathers. Standing there for a while, he found a fairy in white appearing as much more feathers covered the mountain.

At first, the little Taoist was excited and the fairy was very kind. Appreciating the unexpected encounter with the little Taoist, the fairy gave him a light purple plant and then left. As the little Taoist was puzzled at the plant in his hands, a giant dragon occurred. The little Taoist was so scared that he nearly passed out.

The dragon opened its massive bloody mouth and shouted at the little Taoist, "You! A nobody! How dare you take that treasure in your hands? That is a magical herb used for detoxifying hundreds of poisons and resurrecting the dead. How could an ordinary person processes it? Drop it down!" With these words, the dragon grabbed the plant. And the little Taoist was awoken from his dream by the scary dragon.

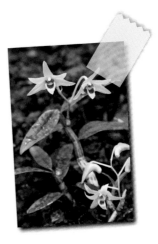

The plant in Taoist's dream is Tie Pi Shi Hu. After learning about the interesting mythological story about Tie Pi Shi Hu, is it more enjoyable when you consume it?

Shi Wei

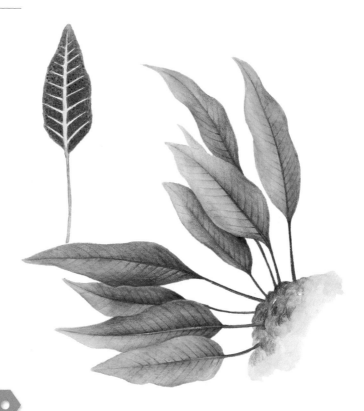

The Secret of the Underside of Shi Wei's Leaves

Shi Wei is a medium-sized epiphytic fern. It can grow up to 30 centimeters in length with its creeping rhizomes and grey-green fronds. If you turn around the leaves, you will find pale brown or brick-red powdery clusters — the sori of Shi Wei where its offspring live.

Chinese Common Names: Shi Pi, Shi Wei, Shi Jian

Latin Name: *Pyrrosia lingua* Farwell

The Origin of Shi Wei

It is said that Sima Qian, the author of *Record of the Grand Historian*, was a royal official whose job was to record the emperor's daily life and important government affairs. Essentially, the emperor permitted Sima Qian to only eulogize his credit while neglect his mistakes. Yet Sima Qian often failed to be compliant and flexible, repeatedly offending the emperor. Worse still, with the revolt ignited by Li Ling, Sima Qian eventually suffered the emperor's brutal torture.

Later, Sima Qian had to seclude himself in mountains and forests, continuing his writing of historical records.

One day, Sima Qian suddenly had difficulty and pain in micturition. He looked down and was freaked out when he found that there was bloody urine. Yet he didn't want to tell it to his daughter and son-in-law. Instead, he consulted the medical book and found that he had suffered from strangury (symptoms such as frequent and urgent urination, scanty urine, urinary pain and heat, etc.).

That day, Sima Qian went alone with a bamboo basket to gather herbs in the mountain. When passing by a small stream, he noticed many primitive and simple ferns growing beside the rocks near the stream. Viewed from a distance, it seemed as if they were growing on the surface of the stones. After consulting the book, he confirmed that these ferns were the medicinal herbs he was searching for. Ancient Chinese people referred to the tanned coating as "Wei" and that is why the plant is called "Shi Wei" in Chinese.

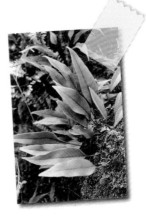

Hu Er Cao

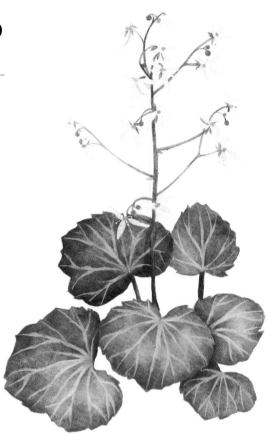

Tips for Planting and Caring Hu Er Cao

1. Hu Er Cao prefers being planted in the shade and requires moisture-regular water with well-drained and rich soil. If growing in a pot, it cannot be exposed to direct sunlight.

2. Hu Er Cao has a strong propagation ability and can propagate in division. Plant it shallowly in the humus soil, tightly press its root, and finally water it.

Chinese Common Names: Shi He Ye, Jin Xian Diao Fu Rong, Lao Hu Er
Latin Name: *Saxifraga stolonifera* Curt.

The Story of Hu Er Cao

One day, a quack came to a village. Although it was quite sultry, he found many villagers' ears stuffed with cotton and some even had pus oozing out. Out of curiosity, he approached a younger to inquire about it.

The younger replied sadly, "Recently, many people have been coughing and getting heat rash and those seriously ill even inflicted ears' discharging pus. Even my sixty-year-old mother has suffered from it and been severely tortured to nearly death."

The quack said to the younger, "I know a treatment that can save your mother."

The younger excitedly brought the quack to his home. After the quack carefully examined the mother's ears, he took some fresh herbs with round leaves and white flowers from his herb collection box and handed them to the younger. He said, "The herb is Hu Er Cao collected from the rocky edge of the mountain behind your village. Take it to decoct for your mother to consume. Reserve a bit to crush and extract juice, then apply it in her ears." With these words, the quack took his leave.

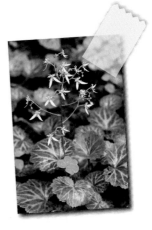

The younger then thanked the quack and quickly decocted the herbs and extracted juice. And his mother consumed it as instructed.

A few days later, his mother didn't feel itchy and there was no pus discharging from her ears. The younger was overjoyed and rushed to tell his neighbors. Then the whole village knew it. After some time, the strange disease gradually disappeared and the village began to come back to life.

Ze Xie

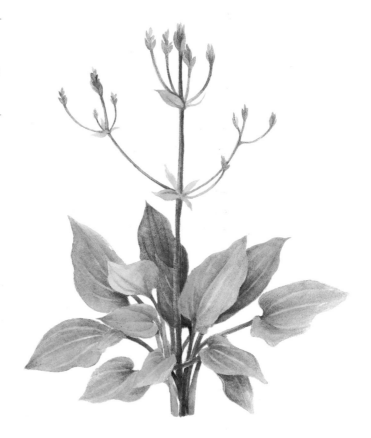

Have you ever heard of Ze Xie?

Although the name sounds a little strange, Ze Xie is a high-valued green plant. It has effects of not only inducing diuresis but also reducing blood lipids.

Its medicinal ingredients, once consumed, will help quickly reduce the cholesterol level in the blood and regulate the level of triglyceride in the blood. Therefore, it is beneficial to balance the level of blood lipids, serving as a natural medicine for preventing arteriosclerosis.

Chinese Common Names: Shui Xie, Mang Yu, Hu Xie
Latin Name: *Alisma plantago-aquatica* L.

The Story of Ze Xie

Once upon a time, a kind girl married a down-to-earth farmer named Ze Xie. They lived a happy life and planted an aquatic plant with white flowers by the pond behind their house.

Unexpectedly, less than half a year after their marriage, Ze Xie was forced to serve in the army. Three years passed without any messages. One day, a fellow villager ran from the battle and told the wife the tragic news that Ze Xie had died on the battlefield. The wife fainted upon hearing the news and the shock worsened her ill health. Six months later, she fell seriously ill with difficulty and pain in micturition and systemic oedema. She lay in the bed on the verge of death.

Ze Xie's wife was aware that she was going to die. In memory of her husband, she called one of her neighbors — Er Jie, to dig up a few plants they had planted together by the pond behind their house. The wife asked the neighbor to decoct the plant with water for her. The neighbor tearfully agreed. To their surprise, the wife recovered after consuming the decoction of the plant with symptoms such as difficulty in micturition and systemic oedema disappearing.

Ze Xie's wife was surprised. She believed that it was the blessing from her husband who encouraged her to live on. From that moment, she regained her spirits and embraced life. In commemoration of her husband, she named this miraculous plant "Ze Xie". That is the origination of the name "Ze Xie" in Chinese.

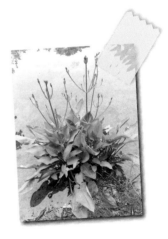

Chang Pu

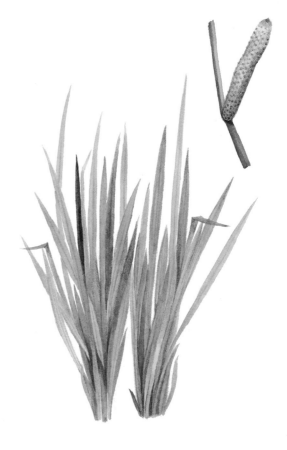

Fun Facts

The Role of Chang Pu in Traditional Festivals

There is a saying that goes, "Place willow branches on gates on the Tomb-sweeping Day and place mugwort on gates on the Dragon Boat Festival." People regard hanging mugwort and Chang Pu (calamus) as an important part of the Dragon Boat Festival. Families will clean the house, place mugwort and Chang Pu on their gates, and hang them on the hall. Why do people hang the plant on the Dragon Boat Festival? In fact, the leaf of Chang Pu looks like a sword. Hanging them at the entrance and bedside symbolizes removing all obstacles, which is a wish for peace and safety for the entire family.

Chinese Common Names: Chou Pu, Ni Chang Pu, Xiang Pu

Latin Name: *Acorus calamus* L.

The Origin of Hanging Chang Pu

Once upon a time, a poor Xiucai's wife named Qing Ying could recite poems and write couplets.

As Qing Ying's home desperately impoverished, she dug some Chang Pu, cleaned them, and hung them on the gate on the fourth day of the fifth lunar month. Moreover, she wrote a poem and posted it beside the gate.

The poem is as follows:

Unfortunate to marry an impoverished man,

For tomorrow's festival, no ritual will be planned.

Do not let the good times slip away,

Just cleanse the Chang Pu with water.

Xiucai felt ashamed at the sight of the poem and then just turned and walked away. On the road, he saw an old ox and decided to sell it to get some money for his wife. However, he was caught by the owner of the ox and was sent to the magistrate of the district.

Interrogated by the magistrate, Xiucai explained everything. The magistrate immediately dispatched a messenger to summon Xiucai's wife.

When Qing Ying came to the court, the magistrate said, "As you can write poems, I require you to write another seven-character quatrain. Once you finish, you will be rewarded with fifty liang of silver ("liang" refers to the ancient monetary unit)."

Upon hearing this, Qing Ying nodded and agreed. She took the brush, ink, and paper and thought for a while. Then she wrote down the four lines:

The rushing Yellow River flows eastward,

Hard to wash away my current shame.

I laugh at myself, not being the Weaving Maid,

How come my husband drags an ox like the Cowherd?

After seeing the poem, the magistrate nodded with approval. He then ordered to give the couple fifty liang of silver and sent them home.

Due to her destitute family, Qing Ying hung the Chang Pu on the Dragon Boat Festival. Yet she unexpectedly received such good fortune. As the news became known, more and more families started hanging the same plant on their doors at every Dragon Boat Festival, which gradually became a folk tradition.

San Bai Cao

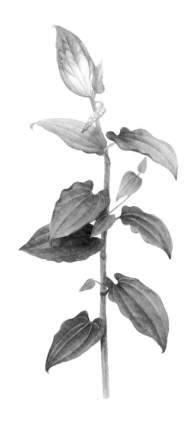

How did ancient people record seasons?

For lack of advanced tools for communication and record in ancient times, people learned to record seasons by observing plants' growth changes. San Bai Cao was one of the plants used to signal phenology. According to the *Compendium of Materia Medica* authored by Li Shizhen, "San Bai Cao grows along ponds and streams and sprouts in March... In April, the leaves on the upper part of the plant will turn white three times... There is a saying that goes: for the first time the leaves turn white, eat wheat; for the second time, eat plums and apricots and for the third time, eat millet." That is to say, when the leaves of San Bai Cao turn white for the first time, it indicates the ripening of wheat; the second time, it signals the ripening of plums and apricots; and the third time, it is time to harvest millet.

Chinese Common Names: Wu Lu Ye Bai, Tang Bian Ou, Bai Hua Lian
Latin Name: *Saururus chinensis* Baill.

The Legend of San Bai Cao

Around 800 years ago, Liu Wansu, a renowned doctor who was over 60 years old, was caught in a storm while he was collecting herbs on the mountain with his apprentices. He fell ill suddenly upon returning home. He had no appetite for food or drinks and suffered from low back soreness with swollen legs. Moreover, he had frequent, urgent and painful urination, which inflicted him a lot. His families and apprentices were confound at this situation when many medicinal decoctions didn't work at all.

At this time, Zhang Yuansu came by as he collected herbs. Upon hearing what happened to Liu Wansu, he quickly went to Liu's house to pay him a visit and gave him a dose of herbs. The herbs looked like *Houttuynia cordata* and Liu Wansu doubted whether it could be used for curing strangury. As he hesitated, one of his apprentices had been decocting the herbs. Liu Wansu realized that the herbs weren't *Houttuynia cordata* when he found that the decoction had a red color with a spicy and fragrant smell. Then he consumed it immediately. After taking it for consecutive three days, his symptoms were relieved and he was finally brought through.

Liu Wansu quickly dispatched someone to invite Zhang Yuansu. He intended to thank him in person and inquire Zhang Yuansu about the magic herbs. Zhang Yuansu took the fresh herbs with three white leaves at the top from his medical box. He said, "The herb was San Bai Cao which grows by ponds or streams with the common name Wetland Lotus Root. It has the effect of clearing heat and inducing urination and removing toxins as well as resolving swelling. Fresh San Bai Cao, without any fishy odor, is similar to *Houttuynia cordata* while the latter has a fishy smell (disappearing when it is dried in the shade). The one previously sent you is dried San Bai Cao." It was quite an eye-opener for Liu Wansu who carefully wrote down the properties, functions and actions of the herb. In his future medical career, he frequently applied it and discovered its amazing effects.

Yue Ji

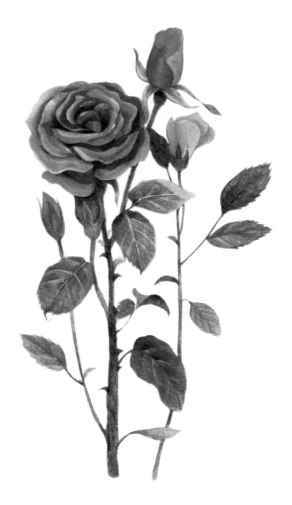

Kids! Do you know what the differences are between rose (*Rosa rugosa* Thunb.) and Yue Ji?

1. Spines. Rose: hard and sharp spines; Yue Ji: flat and sparse spines.

2. Leaves. Rose: depressed, corrugated and lacklustre leaves; Yue Ji: flat and shiny upper surface of leaves.

3. Flowers. Rose: the petals display relatively on the same plane; Yue Ji: the petals display in various planes.

Chinese Common Names: Yue Yue Hong, Yue Yue Hua, Si Ji Hua
Latin Name: *Rosa chinensis* Jacq.

Legend of the Queen of Flowers — Yue Ji

One day, when it was the Queen Mother's birthday, she invited various celestial beings to attend the party in the Heavenly Palace. The Yue Ji fairy collected a basket of Yue Ji as a birthday gift for the Queen Mother. Along the way, she found a scenic place with a green mountain and lush water. Feeling like having fun, she decided to enjoy herself on the mountain.

After a while, she came to realize the Queen Mother's birthday and hurried back to where her flower basket had been placed. "Oh! God!" the fairy shouted as she found that Yue Ji had sprouted. She intended to pull the flowers out but got pricked by the thorns. Regretfully, she could do nothing but return to the Heavenly Palace. All the celestial beings were presenting their gifts to the Queen Mother. It was seen that a profusion of flowers was blooming brightly in the Jade Pool. Seeing Yue Ji fairy, the Queen Mother realized the absence of Yue Ji. She then asked the fairy, "Where are your Yue Ji?" The fairy nervously knelt and explained what had happened. The Queen Mother was enraged and scolded the fairy, "Ah! Audacious fairy! You are too indulgent of fun! Guard! Send her out of the South Gate of Heaven to the mortal realm."

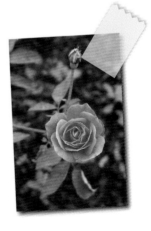

When the Yue Ji fairy came down to the mortal realm, she found Yue Ji and met a laborious man with whom she fell in love at first sight. Later, she married the young man. Since then, the couple carefully nurtured the flowers. Thanks to her good care, the plant bloomed beautifully with colorful flowers. For Yue Ji blooms every month, it's universally adored and gradually becomes popular nationwide.

Lian

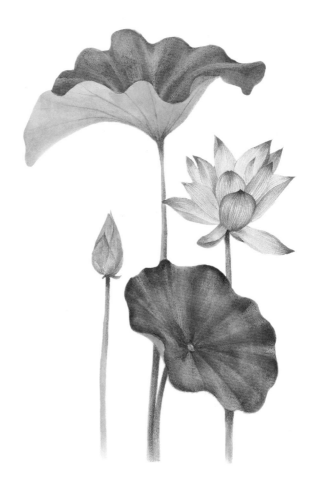

Knowledge about Lian

Lian is also named He in Chinese. Every part of Lian is useful. It's roots and seeds are eatable. Its seed, rhizome, rhizome node, leaf, flower, plumule, etc. can be used as medicine. It has been cultivated and consumed in China for centuries, making China the world's leading producer of it.

Chinese Common Names: Fu Rong, Lotus Root, Lotus
Latin Name: *Nelumbo nucifera* Gaertn.

The Legend of Lian

Long ago, the area along the Jun River was sparsely populated. There lived an uncle with his surname Zhang, who earned his livelihood by fishing. He had no spouse but adopted a son who was one year old.

One day, when Uncle Zhang was out fishing, he suddenly saw a bamboo shoot with a baby crying inside emerging above the river. He carefully retrieved the bamboo tube and opened it, only to find an exceptionally adorable baby girl. Uncle Zhang was delighted and decided to take her in as his own.

As time went by, the two kids grew up. By the time they reached seventeen to eighteen years old, the brother became handsome and the sister was lovely. Especially as for the sister, her rosy cheeks resembled the lotus just rising out of the water, as beautiful as a fairy descending to the mortal realm.

Nobody knew that the baby girl was Lian fairy who was penalized for her mistake and was sent to the mortal realm by the Jade Emperor.

One midnight, celestial troops and generals with their arms descended to the human world, urging the fairy to return to the Heavenly Palace. Appreciated for Uncle Zhang's care, she could not help weeping, with tears falling into the water where a carpet of lotus flowers emerged. Then she bit her finger to write a few words on a handkerchief. As she dropped it, the fairy left with celestial troops and generals.

When daylight came, Uncle Zhang woke up and found that his daughter was gone. He hurried outside, only to see that the clear pond was filled with lotus flowers, with a handkerchief placed by the pond. As a result of divination, Uncle Zhang learned that Lian fairy had descended to the mortal realm. The fairy expressed her gratitude for his care and promised to repay his kindness in the future. She told Uncle Zhang that if he missed her, he could look at the lotus flowers in front of the door, as they were her incarnations.

Bu Gu Zhi

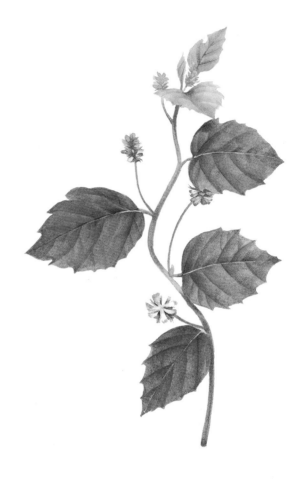

Why Bu Gu Zhi can be used as medicine even though it is poisonous?

It's often said, "Every medicine has its side effects." Although Bu Gu Zhi is poisonous, it is beneficial for tonifying yang. Therefore, we should follow the medical instructions when consuming it. Moreover, it is good medicine for treating vitiligo. To prevent side effects, sunlight or long-wave ultraviolet (UV) irradiation is needed if we take it. Meanwhile, we should take proper eye protection measures to prevent UV damage. It is advisable to take the medicine in the evening and wear protective UV glasses within 24 hours of taking the medicine.

Chinese Common Names: Po Gu Zhi, He Lan Xian, Hu Leek (it looks like the leek gathered from areas of Hu.)

Latin Name: *Cullen corylifolium* Medik.

The Legend of Bu Gu Zhi

It is said that during the Yuanhe period (806-820 AD) of the Tang Dynasty, the 75-year-old prime minister Zheng Yu was appointed by the emperor as the military governor of Hainan. Despite his old age and declining health, Prime Minister Zheng had to rush to take up his new position without any delay. However, due to fatigue caused by the long journey and the unfamiliar environment, he felt exhausted and extremely weak all over as if he were on the verge of death. And he had to be confined to bed. As he was unable to recover, he couldn't attend to state affairs. To cure him, his entourage sent for numerous doctors and Prime Minister Zheng took various medicines, but to no avail.

Later, Mr. Li from the state of He Ling came to Zheng's home three times to recommend the traditional Chinese medicine "Bu Gu Zhi". The prime minister wanted to give it a shot and then followed Li's instruction to take the medicine. After seven to eight days of consumption, it seemed that the medicine worked. Then the prime minister continued taking it for another ten days and he found that the weariness of the body dissolved.

Later, Zheng Yu often took the medicine. When he retired at the age of 82 and returned to Chang'an (the capital of the Tang Dynasty), he was in good physical condition. Then he promoted the medicine and wrote a poem for it:

Seven years as the envoy to land remote,

Only to be told the medicine's unique role.

For it ensures perpetual prime,

Young ladies, don't let white beard bring you dismay.

Since then, it has become known to all that Bu Gu Zhi has the effect of warming the kidney and tonifying yang.

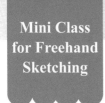
Tips for drawing plants and fruits

To express our gratitude for the support from freehand sketching lovers, this book delivers freehand sketching mini classes and invites the popular illustrator Le Maoxian to tell us in detail how to draw a medicinal plant Gua Lou (*Trichosanthes kirilowii*). What are you waiting for? Let's pick up a pen to draw the beautiful medicinal plant with Le Maoxian!

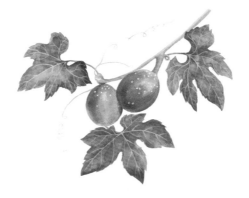

Materials Needed

60-colors water-soluble colored pencils

Solid watercolor paints

Watercolor brushes

300 g hot press watercolor paper

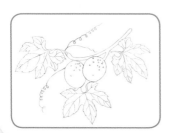

1. Sharpen the colored pencils and gently sketch the contour of Gua Lou. Pay attention to the variations of the lines while drawing. As the fruits of the plant are round in shape, you can draw a circle to establish its shape. Then, proceed to draw leaves in different angles and poses.

206

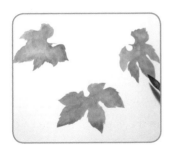

2. Next, paint the leaves with grass green solid watercolor paint as its background color. Blend dark green to delineate the shadow of the leaf edges. Try to keep the strokes clean and crisp, avoid repeated layering.

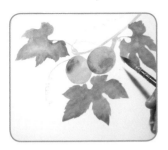

3. Paint the fruits with orange solid watercolor paint as the background color and pay attention to the shadow and the ombre effect of the shadow side. Hit by the light, the upward facing planes tend to be lighter while the shadow side is deeper with a greenish ambient color. Then delineate the vines of the plant. After that, you can use water-soluble colored pencils in the following processes.

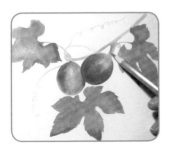

4. Start painting for a second time to emphasize the details of the main part and see the interplay of light and shadow. Deepen the dark side of vines to strengthen the overall volume of Gua Lou.

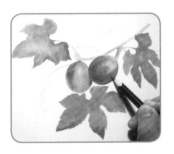

5. Use reddish orange-colored pencils to deepen the terminator of fruits, brown-colored pencil to depict the shadows among fruits, and orange colored pencil to emphasize the transitional surfaces of fruits. Switch to different colored pencils to adjust the color layers of the vines. Always keep the middle orange fruits as the visual center.

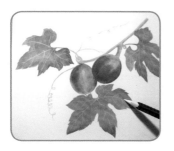

6. Observe the direction of the veins and start outlining them from the center and gradually work outward with a white colored pencil. Notice the plant's proximity when painting to provide areas closer to the line of sight with richer details.

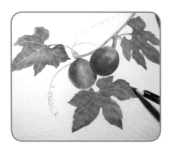

7. Then depict the details of its leaves. Owing to the light, we should pay attention to the color transition from dark at the edge to lighter at the center.

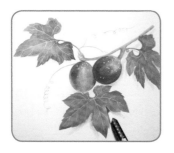

8. Depict some small details such as the color changes at the edges of the leaves. In this way, we will create a more layered visual effect.

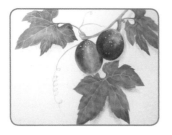

9. Lastly, apply silver and grey colored pencils to add the shadow of Gua Lou, making its leaves and fruits stand vividly revealed on the paper.